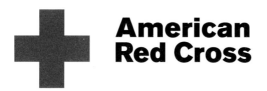

American Red Cross

DOG FIRST AID

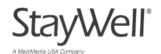

A MediMedia USA Company

Dedication

This book and DVD set is dedicated to man's—and woman's—best friend, who, since primitive times, has been our helper, partner and loyal companion. May we continue to always bring out the best in one another.

Note to Our Readers

No matter how sweet their disposition under normal circumstances, all dogs have the instinct to bite when frightened, injured or threatened. So **always protect yourself by muzzling your dog** before providing first aid, especially if what you need to do might cause more pain. If you cannot safely capture and restrain an injured animal, call your local animal control officer for assistance.

There is a very low risk of transmitting infection between humans and dogs. However, the use of nonlatex, disposable gloves is recommended when treating dog wounds to keep the wound clean. This is not absolutely necessary so do not delay providing care to your dog if gloves are not available.

The editors agreed that "it" is not an appropriate pronoun for a dog. So, to avoid awkward and wordy "he or she" and "him or her" sentence constructions, we alternated the gender reference throughout the text.

When you see this DVD icon in the book margins ◎, it means the skill is demonstrated or the topic is covered in greater detail on the enclosed DVD.

Printing/Binding by RR Donnelly, Spanish Fork

StayWell
780 Township Line Rd.
Yardley, PA 19067

Library of Congress Cataloging-in-Publication Data

Dog first aid.
    p. cm.
  ISBN 978-1-58480-401-7
  1. Dogs—Wounds and injuries—Treatment. 2. Dogs—Diseases—Treatment.
  3. First aid for animals.

SF991.D64 2008
636.7'08960252—dc22

                              2008021672

ISBN 13: 978-1-58480-401-7
09 10/9 8 7 6 5 4 3

About the American Red Cross

Mission of the American Red Cross

The American Red Cross, a humanitarian organization led by volunteers and guided by its Congressional Charter and the Fundamental Principles of the International Red Cross Movement, will provide relief to victims of disaster and help people prevent, prepare for and respond to emergencies.

The American Red Cross helps people prevent, prepare for and respond to emergencies. Last year, almost a million volunteers and 35,000 employees helped victims of almost 75,000 disasters; taught lifesaving skills to millions; and helped U.S. service members separated from their families stay connected. Almost 4 million people gave blood through the Red Cross, the largest supplier of blood and blood products in the United States. The American Red Cross is part of the International Red Cross and Red Crescent Movement. An average of 91 cents of every dollar the Red Cross spends is invested in humanitarian services and programs. The Red Cross is not a government agency; it relies on donations of time, money, and blood to do its work.

Fundamental Principles of the International Red Cross and Red Crescent Movement

Humanity

Impartiality

Neutrality

Independence

Voluntary Service

Unity

Universality

Acknowledgments

This *Dog First Aid* book and DVD set was developed and produced through the combined efforts of the American Red Cross and StayWell. Without the commitment to excellence of both paid and volunteer staff, this product could not have been created.

The American Red Cross and StayWell thank: Alternatives NY, Advertising and Design Agency; Pat Brown, St. Louis Area Chapter; Christine McLaughlin, writer; Lenny Southam, DVM, MPH Veterinary Medical Assistance Team, Chester County Animal Response Team; David Spagnolo, cover photographer; Todd Trice, photographer; Karen Walton, Karen's K-9 Care; and Vickie Wooters, Wooters Dog Training for their contributions to the production of this book and DVD.

The American Red Cross and StayWell also thank the following individual who provided expert review of the materials and support for *Dog First Aid*:

Deborah C. Mandell, VMD, DACVECC
Staff Veterinarian, Emergency Medicine
Adjunct Assistant Professor
Section of Critical Care
Matthew J. Ryan Veterinary Hospital of the University of Pennsylvania
Philadelphia, Pennsylvania

Table of Contents

Table of Contents

Foreword

I smile when I recall how quickly my first dog, Gidgette, would pull the fussy bows off her ears and shake them with all the ferocity her tiny body could muster after returning from the groomers. But it was also upsetting to watch our sweet, playful, longhaired dachshund suffer from epileptic seizures. So my appreciation of the human-animal bond is vividly colored by my personal experiences.

Dogs became integral to our human family ever since their primitive ancestors became domesticated more than 100,000 years ago. Studies have repeatedly shown that their nonjudgmental, unconditional devotion can impart real physical and psychological health benefits to their owners. Beyond that, working dogs, such as K-9, search and rescue, service and therapy dogs, assist countless people. Dogs can make the difference between companionship and loneliness, disability and functionality and, in some cases, even between life and death. We can never fully repay the debt we owe to dogs. That's why I've dedicated my life to helping them—to being their advocate and friend.

As an emergency and critical care veterinarian, I have seen many types of emergencies. I am always deeply touched by the intense feelings people have for their pets. And I have seen cases in which pet owners' quick actions made a huge difference in the health and safety of their pets.

That's why I am very proud to work with the American Red Cross to bring you *Dog First Aid*. This book will serve not only as a handy first aid reference guide, but also will help you identify disease symptoms earlier. Dogs want to be at their best for us and are notorious for hiding illness until the disease is very advanced. But if you learn how to spot subtle changes early, your dog's veterinarian will have a better chance of treating the problem. As with most things in life, being prepared is more than half of the battle.

Wishing you many happy, healthy years with your canine friend,

Deborah C. Mandell, VMD Dipl ACVECC

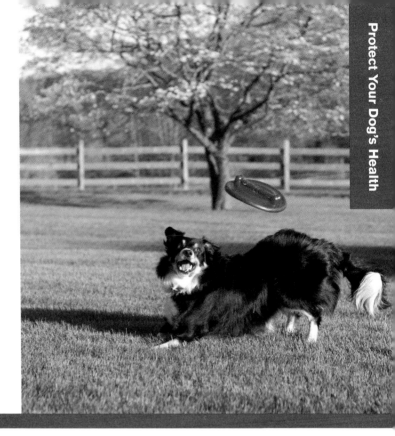

1

Protect Your Dog's Health

You bought this book because you are obviously concerned about your dog's welfare and want to be prepared for health emergencies that might arise from sudden illness or injury. The same responsibility that inspires you to help your dog when something goes wrong is equally important in ensuring his life is full of good health and happiness. In return for your time, love and care, your furry friend will enrich your life immeasurably.

Keep Your Dog Healthy
Take Your Pet to a Vet

Regardless of how or at what age you acquire your dog, be sure to schedule a health check-up with a veterinarian as soon as possible. He or she will make sure your dog receives all the necessary vaccinations and has the proper tests and preventive medications for heartworm and other parasites.

It is crucial to keep your pet's vaccinations up to date. Puppies require a series of inoculations. Take your adult dog to the veterinarian at least yearly.

Your pet's veterinarian is also a great source for advice on training. Do not hesitate to discuss any behavior concerns you may have or to ask for the names of dog trainers in your area.

Provide Good Daily Care

Proper diet and exercise will help you keep your pet lively and trim

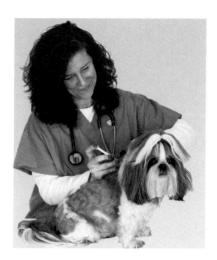

throughout her life. And be sure your pet is groomed regularly.

Proper Diet. Feed your dog the proper amount and type of food. Choose a well-balanced, name-brand or premium-brand dog food that is appropriate for your dog's stage of life. Avoid generic foods because they may not be held to the same rigorous quality standards. Consult your veterinarian about an appropriate diet for your dog.

Always provide your pet with an adequate supply of clean water, and change it frequently.

Regular Exercise. Exercise is essential for your dog. The amount needed depends on the breed, age and any underlying medical conditions he may have. Adequate exercise is always beneficial; it can decrease destructive behavior, as well as keep your pet in good physical shape and make him more satisfied with life indoors. For everyone's health and safety—dogs and people alike—please pick up and dispose of your dog's waste.

Safe, Comfortable Environment. All dogs should be indoor companions, living as members of a family. It's simply not fair to leave a dog alone in the yard most of the time, and it's worse to chain a dog outside for long periods of time. Such dogs often become aggressive and dangerous.

Also, don't allow your dog to roam outside on her own. Your pet might be hit by a car, be injured by other animals, eat poisonous materials, bite someone, contract and spread diseases (including rabies), get lost or stolen or become a victim of abuse.

Put a sticker on the front door or front window of your home to alert others that a pet is inside in the event of an emergency. You can order a free pet rescue sticker from the American Society for the Prevention of Cruelty to Animals at *www.aspca.org.*

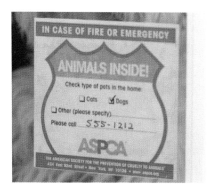

Good Grooming. Brush and comb your pet's coat regularly to keep it healthy and free of matted hair. Ask a veterinarian to show you how to safely clip your pet's nails and care for his ears. Regular grooming will also help you detect skin problems and parasites such as fleas and ticks early. (See pages 95–96 for information on tick removal.)

Dogs with fleas often bite and scratch themselves excessively. If you notice this behavior, look for evidence of fleas. If your pet has fleas, you may actually see the fleas or see flea dirt—tiny black specks that turn reddish when moistened. Talk to your veterinarian about how to treat your pet and your pet's environment safely. (See Fleas, page 91.)

Socialization

A good dog is a socialized dog. Socializing your dog can enhance not just your dog's life, but yours too. A properly socialized dog will behave well in any group or environment and is a great houseguest, hotel guest and outdoor-restaurant partner.

It's best to begin socializing your dog while he is still a puppy. Take him to puppy classes to become accustomed to being around other dogs. Take him on walks in parks and to other public areas where he is likely to encounter a wide variety of people—including children. Allow friendly interaction when it seems safe and appropriate.

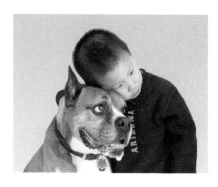

tips

PESTICIDE DOs AND DON'Ts

Do—
1. Read all labels and follow directions carefully.
2. Make sure insecticides are safe to use in combination if using more than one product, such as—
   - A flea collar and a dip.
   - More than one kind of flea insecticide.
   - Professional exterminator chemicals used around the home.
3. Talk to your veterinarian about how to treat your pet and her environment safely.

Don't—
1. Use a product more frequently, in higher concentrations or in a larger quantity than directed on the label.
2. Use a product for an age group or animal not specifically mentioned on the label.
3. Use pesticides on extremely young or old, sick, pregnant or heartworm-infected animals.

Regardless of how well trained or socialized your dog is, never leave a young child alone with him or allow anyone to hurt your dog.

If you acquire an adult dog, take him to a professional dog trainer (you can ask your veterinarian for suggestions) and ask the trainer to evaluate your dog's behavior around other dogs and people.

If there are off-leash dog parks nearby and your dog is friendly and enjoys them, take him there on a regular basis. Dog parks encourage healthy socialization and are appropriate for most dogs. Most dog parks prohibit aggressive dogs.

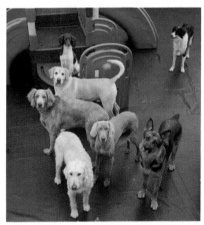

To Crate or Not to Crate
A crate is a metal or plastic portable cage just large enough to contain the dog. The practice of using this cage for training purposes—usually housebreaking—is known as crating. Because a dog will not soil her sleeping area if she can possibly avoid it, crate training a puppy makes

housebreaking easier. If you plan to crate train your puppy, make sure the crate is not so large that the puppy can relieve herself at one end and sleep at the other. If you buy a crate sized for an adult dog, block off part of it until your puppy grows into it.

Use the crate judiciously. Make sure it is large enough for your dog to lie down, stand up and turn around in comfortably. Also, make sure your dog gets ample family play time and affection when outside of her crate and do not force her to spend an excessive amount of time isolated away from your family. If your dog sleeps in her crate, put the crate in your bedroom when you turn in for the night. A dog that feels safe and comfortable in a crate will be easier to transport in a car or on an aircraft or to evacuate in a disaster.

Spaying and Neutering
Pet overpopulation is like a disease—it kills millions of dogs each year. But there is a cure: spaying (for females) or neutering (for males). This cure also has health and behavioral benefits for your pet. The American Veterinary Medical Association and others agree it is safe to spay or neuter most puppies as early as 8 weeks of age.

When performed early, spaying can prevent breast cancer (mammary tumors). Spaying at any age eliminates the risk of uterine infections, uterine or ovarian cancer and some skin disorders. Neutering can pre-

vent testicular disease and greatly lessen the risk of prostate disease.

Pets who are spayed or neutered are generally better, more affectionate companions, and neither you nor your pet needs to suffer through the physical and behavioral problems associated with heat cycles. Spayed or neutered pets are less likely to roam, spray or mark territory or be aggressive. In many studies of serious dog bites, evidence shows that bites are more often inflicted by unneutered dogs.

NOTE:
- **It is not better for your female pet's health to delay spaying until after her first heat or to let her have a litter before spaying.**
- **Neutering will not affect a dog's instinct to protect his human family.**
- **Spayed or neutered pets do not automatically become fat and lazy.**

ID—Your Lost Pet's Ticket Home
Even though your pet should live indoors and remain under your supervision when outside, pets should wear collars and up-to-date identification at all times.

If your pet becomes lost, a tag with your name, address and phone number can help reunite you and your pet. But regardless of the type of ID on your pet, search for your lost pet immediately. Contact local animal shelters and pet stores, put up signs and call all surrounding veterinarians and the police.

If all else fails, visit these lost pet Web sites:

- Fido Finder: *www.fidofinder.com*
- Lost Pet SOS: *www.lostpetsos.org*
- Find That Pet: *www.findthatpet.com*

How to ID Your Pet

Follow these tips to make sure your dog has proper ID at all times:

- Affix license or rabies tags to your pet's collar as required by state or local law.
- Add a tag with essential medical information for pets with medical problems.
- Attach a temporary tag when traveling with your pet, with a contact name and phone number of where you'll be staying.
- For back-up ID, have an ID number permanently tattooed on your pet, and register the number with a recognized national organization such as The National Dog Registry (800-NDR-DOGS or e-mail *info@natldogregistry.com*) or at Tatoo-A-Pet (800-TATTOOS or e-mail *info@tattoo-a-pet.com*).
- Or consider having a microchip implanted under your pet's skin by a veterinarian or animal shelter. The microchip—about the size of a grain of rice—contains a code that a scanner can detect and read. Always register your pet's microchip with the national database.

Traveling With Your Pet

Your dog will be happier if allowed to accompany you when you travel. However, you must always balance this need against his overall health and safety. If you are moving to a new area, of course you will take your pet with you. You simply need to consider the best and safest mode of travel for your dog. However, if you're thinking about taking your pet on vacation with you, you must consider your pet's overall health, whether your pet likes to travel, where you'll be staying, the time of year, your options if you don't take your pet and whether taking your pet on a vacation is really in his best interest.

If traveling abroad, be aware that some countries have requirements that can take up to 6 to 8 months to complete, so start planning as early as possible.

Have your pet examined by your veterinarian before any trip. Get any required legal travel documents (contact the airline as well); make sure vaccinations are up to date and get any medications your pet might need. Medications used specifically for travel should be given to your pet on a trial basis several days before you leave to make sure your pet doesn't suffer adverse effects.

In the Car
When riding in the car—

- Your dog should be in a crate or carrier or restrained in a special harness that attaches to the seat belt. If you use a pet barrier in the back seat or deck of your SUV, be sure it is sturdy and firmly attached so it does not collapse on your pet.
- Your dog should never ride in the front passenger seat, especially one that is airbag equipped.
- Never let your pet out of the car without proper restraint.
- Don't let your dog ride with his head out the window; he could be hurt by flying debris.

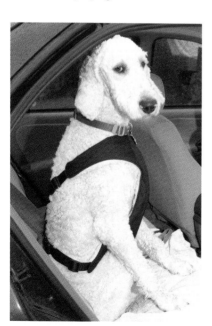

- On a long trip, take your pet's travel kit (see What to Pack for Your Pet, page 8). Keep a supply of water in the car and be prepared to make frequent rest stops.
- Never leave your pet alone in a parked car, not even for a few moments. He will be vulnerable to heat distress or theft.

On a Plane
Although thousands of pets fly on airlines without problems, there are risks. Follow these tips:

- Don't fly your pet unless it's absolutely necessary.
- If you must take your pet when you fly, make travel arrangements well in advance and ask about all regulations, including any quarantine requirements at your destination.
- If you have a small pet, arrange to carry her onboard with you.
- If your pet must travel in the cargo area—
    - Use a direct flight.
    - Travel on the same flight as your pet.
    - Ask to watch your pet being loaded and unloaded.
    - When you board, notify the captain and at least one flight attendant that your pet is in the cargo hold.

On a Boat
If your pet *enjoys* going sailing or fishing with you, here are some tips to help you ensure his safety and comfort:

- Take a generous supply of drinking water for your dog, and teach him to drink out of a sports bottle to prevent spills.
- Provide a shady retreat where your dog can escape the sun.
- Make sure your dog has a well-fitted, brightly colored canine personal flotation device (available in marine-supply stores), and take him out for a trial swim with it ahead of time to make sure it provides enough buoyancy. Most have handles that will help you lift your dog out of the water. Make sure the attachment straps are comfortable and will not cut into his skin.
- If you have a large boat, teach your dog to relieve himself in a specific spot that is easy for you to clean. Otherwise, take him back to land for regular pit stops, and be sure to clean up his waste when you do.
- Try a short trip first, and if your dog is prone to seasickness or acts distressed while aboard your boat, make other arrangements for your pet while you enjoy boating.

NOTE: Not all dogs can swim. Moreover, very lean and well-muscled dogs are not buoyant and will tire quickly while swimming.

What to Pack for Your Pet

Here are some essentials to take when you travel with your pet or if you must evacuate with your pet in a disaster:

- Medications and medical records
- Food and bowls
- First aid kit
- Bedding
- Leash, collar and tags
- Grooming supplies
- Current pet photo that includes you (in case your pet gets lost)
- A favorite toy or two
- A sturdy, well-ventilated carrier

For more information on what to pack in case of a disaster, see Be Prepared for Disaster, page 19.

If you choose to leave your pet behind while you go on vacation,

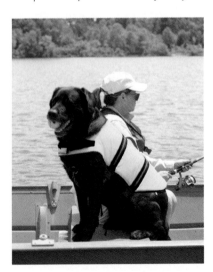

be sure whoever is caring for your pet has your vacation phone number, complete feeding and care instructions and the number of your veterinarian. It is also a good idea to tell your veterinarian who will be caring for your pet and what your wishes are for veterinary care in case of emergency while you're gone.

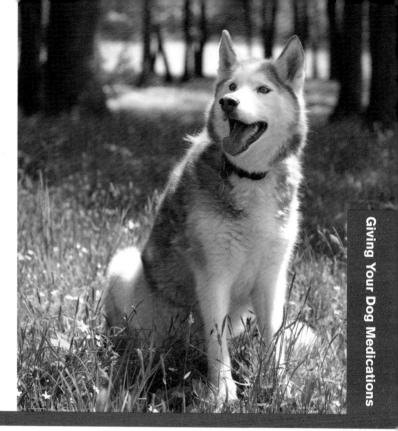

2

Giving Your Dog Medications

It's not a simple task to give your dog medicine, especially pills, but you'll probably have to do it at some point in your dog's life. But following the steps provided in this chapter is a foolproof way to ensure your dog is on his way back to good health. It's important to remember never to give medications by mouth to an animal who is lying down, unconscious, vomiting, having trouble breathing, having a seizure or to one that is acting aggressively.

Administering Eye Medications
Technique

1. Rest the side of the hand that you will use to administer the medication on the bone above your dog's upper eyelid. This will help prevent poking the medication tube into the eye if you are jostled.
2. Tilt the head backward slightly with the palm of your other hand under the chin supporting the head.
3. With this same hand, pull down the lower eyelid with your thumb.
4. Place drops or ointment directly in the eye with enough distance to ensure the tip of the dispenser does not touch the eye.

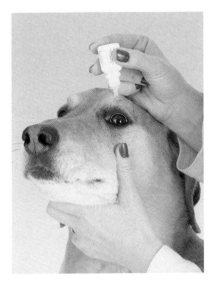

Administering Ear Medications
Technique

1. Stand on the same side of the animal as the ear you will be treating.
2. If the dog is floppy-eared, lift the floppy portion so you can clearly see inside the ear opening.
3. Place the drops or ointment in the middle of the ear opening.
4. Rub or massage the base of the ear to allow the medication to drop down into the deeper portions of the ear.

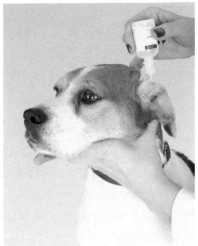

Liquids

For many people, giving liquid medication to a pet is easier than giving pills. Keep a baby dosing syringe or cyedropper (both with measurements marked), which can be found in pharmacies or in the baby section of grocery stores, in your pet first aid kit (see Pet First Aid Kit, page 18).

Here are some common conversions you may find helpful for correct dosing:

- 1 milliliter (ml) = 1 cc
- 5 cc = 1 teaspoon
- 15 cc = 1 tablespoon
- 8 ounces = 1 cup

Technique

1. Place the end of the eyedropper or syringe on one side of your dog's mouth, just behind the pointy canine teeth, where the teeth are shortest and flattest.
2. Gently position the dropper above the lower teeth, or in the pouch between the gums and lower teeth. (Placing the medicine over the teeth will result in less spitting of the medicine than placing it in the pouch.)
3. Slowly administer the medication, giving it no faster than the animal can swallow.

IMPORTANT: Never give your pet any medications unless they are prescribed by a veterinarian.

Pills and Capsules
Technique

1. With one hand, hold your pet's upper jaw toward the ceiling by taking hold of the snout and gently pointing it upward. This will cause the lower jaw to drop slightly.
2. With the other hand, gently pull down on the very front-most part of the lower jaw.
3. Place the tablet in the center of the back of the tongue, as far back into the mouth as you safely can.
4. Hold the mouth closed once you have given the pill until your pet swallows or licks her nose. Sometimes gently blowing on the nose or rubbing the throat will cause the animal to swallow.

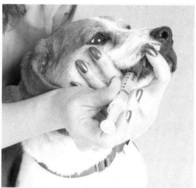

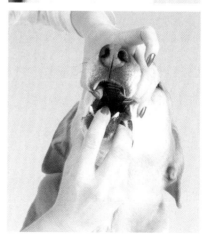

Giving Your Dog Medications

Pills can also be hidden in food, but you must ensure your pet does not eat the morsel and spit out the pill. Peanut butter works well because it is sticky and tends to hold the tablet. If your dog is vomiting or has diarrhea, hiding medication in food is not a good idea because it may make the condition worse.

There are also commercial pill "guns" available. These plastic tubes hold the pill and allow you to place it in the back of the throat without putting your hands in the animal's mouth.

NOTE: It may be easier to give your dog medication by having him in a sitting position backed into a corner, so he can't get up.

Topical Ointments and Creams

Compared with administering pills, ointments and creams are a dog walk in the park. While wearing disposable, nonlatex gloves, apply the medication in a thin layer. However, the most important thing to remember is to keep your dog from licking the ointment, as it will lessen its effectiveness and might even give her an upset stomach. You might consider putting an Elizabethan collar on your dog to prevent her from licking the medication. Or, depending on where the wound is, you might also consider putting one of your old T-shirts or boxer shorts on her to cover the affected area.

Elizabethan Collars (E-Collars)

These collars are designed for function, not fashion. And they're extremely helpful in keeping your dog from aggravating a wound, biting sutures or licking off ointments and creams. Your dog may act a little hesitant at first and may bang into walls and furniture due to lack of peripheral vision, but it's only temporary, and he'll eventually forgive you, especially when he feels better. You can purchase an Elizabethan collar from any pet supply store or from your veterinarian.

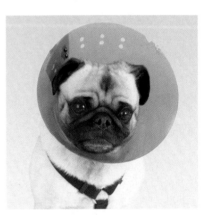

Adverse Reactions From Human Food and Medicines

Dogs should never be given human food or medicines unless prescribed by the veterinarian.

On the next page is a partial list of foods and medicines to keep away from your dog. Consult with your veterinarian for a more specific list of foods that are harmful to your dog.

Foods
- Alcoholic beverages (all types, including beer)
- Avocado
- Bones from chicken, fish (and other meat bones a chewing dog can break apart or splinter) – these can cause choking, get stuck in the esophagus or stomach or puncture internal organs.
- Chives
- Chocolate and cocoa (all forms)
- Coffee and other caffeinated beverages (all forms)
- Garlic
- Macadamia nuts
- Milk
- Mushrooms
- Onions, onion powder
- Raisins and grapes
- Salt
- Xylitol sweetened products (typically found in sugar-free gum)
- Yeast dough

Medicines
Even small doses of some human medications can be lethal to your pet. Some of these include:

- Antidepressants
- Anticancer drugs
- Cold medicines
- Diet pills
- Pain killers (including aspirin, ibuprofen (Advil®, Motrin® Nurofen®), naproxen (Naprosyn®) and acetaminophen or paracetamol (Tylenol®))
- Vitamins (particularly those that contain iron)

In addition, many plants and household products are poisonous to your pet. For more information, visit the American Society for the Prevention of Cruelty to Animals (ASPCA) Web site at *www.aspca.org* and scroll down to "Animal Poison Control" in the Expert Advice menu on the left.

If you suspect that your pet has eaten a poisonous substance call the ASPCA National Animal Poison Control Center at 888-4ANI-HELP (888-426-4435) immediately. There is a charge for the consultation. In critical cases, the center will do as many follow-up calls as necessary and will contact your veterinarian at your request.

3

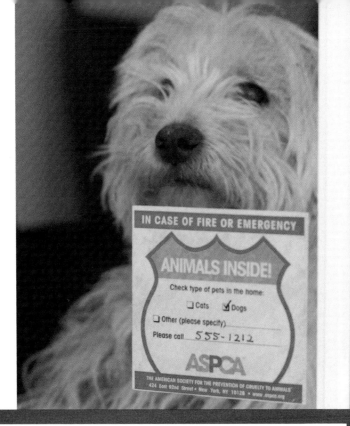

IN CASE OF FIRE OR EMERGENCY

ANIMALS INSIDE!

Check type of pets in the home:

☐ Cats ☑ Dogs

☐ Other (please specify)

Please call 555-1212

ASPCA

THE AMERICAN SOCIETY FOR THE PREVENTION OF CRUELTY TO ANIMALS®
424 East 92nd Street • New York, NY 10128 • www.aspca.org

Be Prepared

In any type of emergency, having supplies before you need them and knowing how to respond can increase the chance of a positive outcome. This is especially true during a regional disaster when help might be delayed and normal supply chains could be cut off. If an evacuation were ordered, would you be ready to pick up and go at a moment's notice? Gather the items listed in this section to complete your dog's first aid and emergency supplies kits. For more information about emergency preparedness for your family, visit *www.redcross.org* and click on Be Red Cross Ready.

Pet First Aid Kit

Every dog owner should have some basic first aid supplies on hand. If your pet has special medical conditions, ask your veterinarian what additional items you should include. Check your kit periodically to replace expired medicines and replenish used supplies. The pet first aid kit can be stored in a small, sturdy box. Consider carrying a smaller version in your car. Remember to keep all medications and medical supplies out of the reach of young children and pets.

A pet first aid kit should include:
- [ ] Absorbent compresses (sometimes called gauze sponges) in assorted sizes
- [ ] Adhesive tape, hypoallergenic
- [ ] Antibiotic ointment (triple, available at pharmacies)
- [ ] Blanket (emergency or "space" blanket)
- [ ] Clean cloth
- [ ] Cold compress
- [ ] Diphenhydramine (Benadryl®) in an appropriate dose for your pet's size if approved by your veterinarian for allergic reactions (see Diphenhydramine Dosing, page 43). Make sure the product contains diphenhydramine ONLY and no other cold or allergy remedies. This will have an expiration date.
- [ ] *Dog First Aid* book
- [ ] Expired credit card (to scrape away stingers)
- [ ] Epsom salts (to make saline solution)
- [ ] Gloves (disposable, nonlatex)
- [ ] Glucose paste or corn syrup (if your pet is diabetic or has a history of low blood sugar)
- [ ] Grooming clippers
- [ ] Hydrogen peroxide, 3 percent (check expiration date)
- [ ] List of emergency telephone numbers, including your pet's veterinarian, an after-hours emergency veterinary hospital and the American Society for the Prevention of Cruelty to Animals' Animal Poison Control Center (1-888-426-4435)
- [ ] Muzzle—A cage muzzle is best, but a soft collapsible one may be more convenient to carry. Get one you know fits your pet. If you do not have a muzzle, have plenty of roll gauze available to create a makeshift muzzle.
- [ ] Nail clippers appropriate for your dog's nails
- [ ] Needle-nose pliers
- [ ] Nylon leash (at least one)
- [ ] Petroleum jelly
- [ ] Penlight
- [ ] Rectal thermometer (non-mercury/non-glass)
- [ ] Roll cohesive wrap, 3-inch width (stretches and clings to itself)
- [ ] Roll gauze, 2-inch width, cotton
- [ ] Rubbing alcohol (isopropyl)
- [ ] Scissors, small, with blunt end
- [ ] Sterile gauze pads, non-adherent (assorted sizes)
- [ ] Sterile, water-based lubricant (such as KY® Jelly) that washes off easily (to keep fur away from a wound you are treating)
- [ ] Syringe (baby dose size)

- ☐ Sterile eye lubricant (available at pharmacies)
- ☐ Sterile saline eye wash (available at pharmacies)
- ☐ Styptic powder (to stop bleeding from broken nails, available at pet stores)
- ☐ Towel
- ☐ Tweezers
- ☐ Wire cutters, small (to cut barb off embedded hooks if you take your dog fishing)

Be Prepared for Disaster

A disaster can strike at any time and anywhere. It is important to know if earthquakes, floods, tornados and severe weather can affect your area, and whether you live in a special hazard area, like a flood plain, wildfire or hurricane-prone area. If you must evacuate in a disaster, use the recommended evacuation routes. Some areas can be dangerous, so avoid shortcuts. In the case of any evacuation, LEAVE EARLY to avoid heavy traffic or gridlock.

Get a Kit

You should assemble an emergency supplies kit ahead of time for everyone in your household, including your pet. Keep everything in sturdy containers (duffel bags, covered plastic storage containers, etc.) that can be carried easily. The kit for your dog should include—

- ☐ Pet identification (see below for more information).
- ☐ A pet first aid kit, including this book, and any medications your pet is taking.

- ☐ Medical records stored in a waterproof container; include vaccination records, your pet's medical conditions, veterinarian's name and phone number and any other special concerns.
- ☐ Food and water for each pet: a 3-day supply for evacuation and a 2-week supply for the home, including a manual can opener, if needed, for canned food.
- ☐ Food bowls.
- ☐ Bedding/blankets and toys to help reduce stress and provide comfort.
- ☐ Leashes, harnesses and carriers to transport your pets safely and to ensure your pets cannot escape. Carriers should be large enough for the animal to stand comfortably, turn around and lie down.
- ☐ Garbage bags, quart-size storage bags, newspapers, paper towels and bleach to make a sanitizing solution for cleaning up pet waste.

Pet Identification Is Extremely Important! Your dog should wear current identification on his collar at all times. In case of a disaster, include an additional temporary tag that lists your out-of-area emergency contact phone numbers. It's also a good idea to have a microchip implanted in your pet beforehand, in case the collar and tags fall off (see How to ID Your Pet, page 6). Be sure to include photos of your pet taken with you to prove your ownership and to help find your pet if he becomes lost.

Make a Plan
Even if you don't live in a flood plain, near an earthquake fault line, in wildfire country or in a coastal area, it's crucial to think about how you will cope. Be aware that "natural disasters" aren't the only emergencies you need to be prepared for. Fire, acts of terrorism and other human-caused disasters, such as a hazardous material spill, could require a prompt response. And remember, if you and your family need to evacuate, so does your pet.

Make a List of Important Phone Numbers. At the top of your emergency preparedness to-do list should be to create a list of important phone numbers. These should include people and organizations in your area, outside of your area and in a different state that you can rely on in the event of a disaster, including your family and friends; pet-friendly hotels; veterinarians/emergency veterinary hospitals; boarding facilities; and, as a last resort, a list of local and remote animal shelters.

Remember that most human emergency shelters will not allow animals, except service dogs, to stay there. Also understand that if you have more than one pet, you might have to house them separately. Thus, it is very impor-

tant to determine ahead of time where you will take your pet in an emergency.

Be Informed
Depending on the type of disaster, you may need to stay at home or follow an order to evacuate. Plan for both possibilities. Listen to the radio and TV, and check the Internet for up-to-date information and promptly follow the authorities' instructions. For more information on how to prepare, visit *www.ready.gov* or call 1-800-BE-READY.

IMPORTANT: At the first sign of an emergency, bring your pet into the house and confine her so you can leave with her quickly. Do not wait until the last minute to gather your supplies. Have your disaster supplies ready to go.

Evacuating With Pets. Call ahead to confirm emergency shelter arrangements for both your family and your pet, whether you're staying together or separately. Be sure your pet and her carrier have up-to-date identification and contact information, including the phone number of your temporary shelter and its location.

If you do evacuate, keep your pet with you or know the designated emergency location where you will take your pet. Animals left inside a home can escape if the home is damaged by storms. Animals left to fend for themselves outside are likely to become victims of exposure, starvation, predators, contaminated food or water, or accidents. Leaving dogs tied or chained outside during a disaster is a death sentence.

Staying Home. If you are at home during a storm, identify a safe area of your home where you can stay with your pet. Remember to keep your dog on a leash or in a carrier, and make sure he is wearing identification. Be sure to have your other emergency supplies handy (see Get a Kit, page 19).

If You're Not Home When Disaster Strikes. Make arrangements in advance with a trusted neighbor who has a copy of your house key. Ask your neighbor to take your pet and meet you at a specified location if a disaster strikes when you're not at home and an evacuation order is issued. Be sure that person is comfortable with your pet and knows where he is likely to be, as well as where your disaster supplies are kept. In addition, have all your contact phone numbers readily available for your neighbor.

Returning Home After the Disaster. Your home could be a very different place when the disaster is over. So wait until authorities say it is safe for you and your dog to return. Once you do, don't allow your dog to roam loose throughout your home. Familiar landmarks and smells might be gone, and she will probably become disoriented.

For a few days, keep your dog on a leash and/or in a carrier inside the house. Finally, be patient with your dog. Try to establish a calming environment and get her back into her normal routines as soon as possible, but be ready for stress-induced behavioral problems. If these persist, or if your pet seems to have health problems, talk to your veterinarian.

Be Prepared

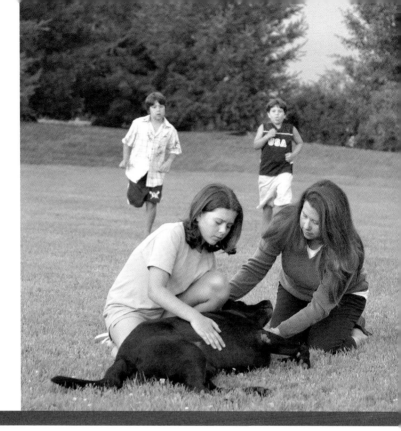

4

How to Know if It's a Medical Emergency

The best way to recognize and respond to an emergency is to know what is normal for your dog and to know how to recognize an emergency. However, if you are unsure about a situation, always call your veterinarian. Many conditions have a better prognosis if caught early. Another important thing to know is that dogs compensate very well for most disease processes, which means that by the time your pet begins showing signs of illness, he may already be in an advanced stage of disease. So take him to a veterinarian as soon as possible.

Know What's Normal

It will be easier to recognize what is abnormal for your pet if you first become familiar with what is normal. Observe how your dog breathes, eats, drinks, walks, urinates and defecates so you will be sensitive to changes that might signal problems.

Check the Scene

Before approaching an injured dog, look around for potential hazards that may still exist and could potentially harm you. For example, if an animal has been struck by a car, make sure there are no other cars approaching before running into the street; or if your dog is in a fight, don't get between the two animals or you might become the next victim.

Check the Dog

Make an initial evaluation that should be completed in about 1 minute. Do the following:

- **Situation.** Quickly observe the animal's body; posture; presence of blood, urine, feces or vomit; breathing pattern; sounds and other materials (possible poisons around the dog).
- **Airway.** Is it open? If not, see Airway, page 36.
- **Breathing.** Is the animal breathing? If not, see Breathing, page 36.
- **Bleeding.** If the animal is bleeding, see Bleeding, page 48.
- **Circulation.** Is there a heartbeat and a pulse? If not, see Circulation, page 37.

- **Mucous membrane color.** See Observe Your Dog's Mucous Membrane Color, page 27.
- **Capillary refill time.** See Capillary Refill Time, page 28.
- **Level of consciousness.** Is the animal alert, awake, seizuring, disoriented, hyperactive, depressed or unconscious? If the animal is seizuring, see Seizures, page 101.

Always have the telephone number of your veterinarian, 24-hour veterinary emergency hospital, American Society for the Prevention of Cruelty to Animals' Animal Poison Control Center (1-888-426-4435) and animal shelter or animal care and control agency readily available!

Heart Rate and Pulse

You can feel your dog's heartbeat at about the point where the left elbow touches the chest (about the fifth rib). **Remember to use a light touch; if you press too hard you will not feel the pulse.**

1. Lay your dog down on her right side. But, if it's easier, allow her to stand.
2. Gently bend the left front leg at the elbow and bring it back to where it touches the chest.
3. Place your hand or a stethoscope (available at most pharmacies) over this area to feel or hear and count heartbeats.

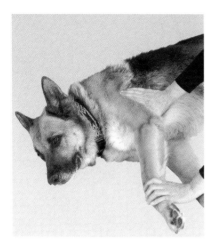

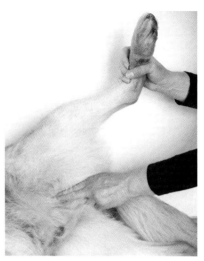

You can feel your dog's pulse by lightly touching your middle and index fingers to these three additional locations.

The Inner Thigh. (This is the easiest of the three locations to feel the pulse.)

1. Lay your dog down, on either side.
2. Gently lift her upper hind leg away from the lower hind leg.
3. Place your two fingers as high up as possible on the inside of either leg, just where the leg meets the body wall.
4. Feel for a recess in the middle of the leg approximately half way between the front and back; this recess is where the blood vessels run and where you will find the pulse.

Just Below the Wrist (Carpus).

1. Have your dog sit or lie down.
2. Locate the area just above the middle pad on the underside of either front paw.
3. Lightly place your middle and index fingers at this point.

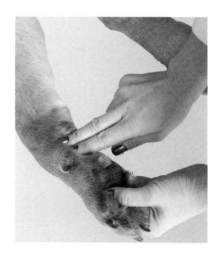

Is It an Emergency?

tips

What's Normal

Normal Heart and Pulse Rates

Heart rates outside these ranges could signal an emergency:

- ☐ Puppy (less than 1 year old): 120–160 beats per minute
- ☐ Small, miniature or toy breed (30 pounds or less): 100–140 beats per minute
- ☐ Medium to large breed (greater than 30 pounds): 60–100 beats per minute

Normal Breathing Rates
- ☐ 10–30 breaths per minute
- ☐ Up to 200 pants per minute (breathing with its mouth open and tongue out)

Normal Temperatures for Dogs
- ☐ A temperature of 100°–102.5° F is normal.
- ☐ A temperature lower than 100° F or greater than 104° F is an emergency; call your veterinarian at once.

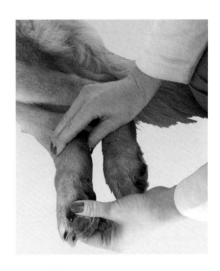

Just Below the Ankle (Hock).
1. Have your dog sit or lie down.
2. Locate the area just below the ankle on the top side of either hind paw.
3. Lightly place your middle and index fingers at this point.

Breathing Rate
1. Have your pet either stand or lie down.
2. Watch your pet and count the number of times that the chest rises and falls in 1 minute.

In an emergency, if you are not sure if your pet is breathing, try one of these techniques:

- Hold a cotton ball or tissue just in front of the nostrils and see if it moves
- Hold a mirror up to your pet's nose and look for condensation

Respiratory Pattern. When a dog inhales normally, the chest should expand. If the abdomen expands instead of the chest, that could indicate a problem. Exhaling should be an easy process with no work involved. If your pet makes loud, shallow or gasping sounds when breathing, or is not breathing, this is an emergency; see CPR, page 36.

How to Take Your Dog's Temperature

1. See Restraint Techniques, page 31.
2. Use a pediatric digital thermometer, found in any drug store.
3. Lubricate the thermometer with a water-based lubricant or petroleum jelly.
4. Insert the tip of the thermometer into the rectum (just beneath the tail).
5. Leave the thermometer inserted until it beeps.
6. Remove and read the number.

Observe Your Dog's Mucous Membrane Color

The color of your dog's mucous membranes (gums and inner eyelids) can help you determine if enough oxygen and blood are flowing to all of his tissues. To check the color of the mucous membranes, lift your dog's upper or lower lip and observe the color of his gums or inner lip.

- If your dog has black (pigmented) mucous membranes, place your thumb on the skin just under the lower eyelid and gently pull down to observe the inner eyelid membrane color. It should be pink, which means the tissues are receiving enough oxygen.
- If your dog's mucous membranes are blue, pale, yellow, cherry red, white, brick red or brown, this is an emergency. Call the veterinarian immediately. If your dog's mucus membranes are any other color, see Poisoning, page 96.

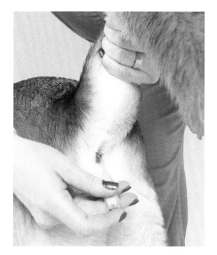

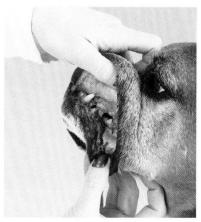

Is It an Emergency?

Capillary Refill Time

Observing how soon the gums or inner lips return to their normal pink color after you press on them is a quick way to know if your dog's blood circulation is normal.

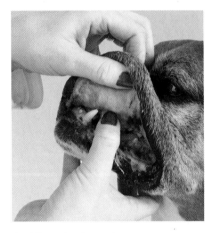

1. After checking the mucous membrane color, press lightly on the gums or inner lip.
2. Observe the color as it turns white and then pink again. The pink color should return after 1 or 2 seconds.
3. Call your veterinarian at once if the pink color returns in less than 1 second or more than 3 seconds. This is an emergency.

How to Approach, Capture and Restrain a Dog

Always approach a sick or injured dog slowly and cautiously. Even your own sweet pooch might strike out if frightened or in pain. Observe her posture and expressions—especially her face, ears, tail, fur and body. Listen to the sounds she's making.

As you approach, allow the animal to smell the back of your hand. Never make quick or jerky movements or loud sounds. Allow the dog to see what you are doing and watch her reactions carefully. Always speak in a soft, soothing tone to an injured or sick animal. Avoid direct eye contact—some dogs may perceive it as a threat.

Body Language Warning Signs

Any of these behaviors may signal that a dog is inclined to bite. Do not attempt treatment on any dog exhibiting any of these warning signs:

- Ears held forward; tail may wag slightly
- Growling and with fur standing up on shoulders, back and hind end
- Snarling with upper lips lifted and teeth exposed

OR. . .

- Crouching with tail between legs
- Ears held straight back or flat against the head
- Snarling and with fur on the back raised

OR. . .

- Assuming submissive posture
  - Lying on his side with belly exposed
  - Making licking gestures or urinating

Even a fearfully submissive dog can quickly become a biting dog if you continue to approach.

If you cannot safely handle an animal, call your local animal shelter or animal care and control agency. You can't help an animal by getting hurt yourself. While waiting for assistance to arrive, you can do other things to help, such as diverting traffic if an animal has been hit by a car and is still in the street, or keeping other people and animals away from the injured animal.

Capture Techniques

Always allow a dog to know where you are so you don't surprise her.

Leash. Leather, nylon or canvas leashes are strong and easy to use. (Do not use chain-link leashes.)

1. Make a large loop in a leash by passing the end you normally connect to a collar through the hole in the handle.
2. Standing just behind or to the side of the animal's head, drop the large loop over the neck and tighten.

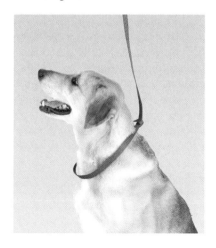

Towel or Blanket. If the dog is small (less than 30 pounds) you can sometimes capture her by dropping a towel or blanket over her.

1. First observe the dog's position so you don't put your hands near her mouth.
2. Drop a large towel or blanket from above and behind the dog.
3. Grasp the scuff of her neck so she cannot turn around and bite your hand through the towel.
4. Transfer the dog to a sturdy box or carrier.

Gloves. While you might think wearing thick work gloves will help you safely handle a dog, they will cause you to lose dexterity, and dogs can bite through most glove material. However, wear nonlatex gloves when treating wounds to prevent the spread of infection.

Muzzle. You can purchase a muzzle at pet stores, veterinary hospitals and through pet catalogs. They come in various sizes and should be part of your pet first aid kit (see Pet First Aid Kit, page 18). Muzzles may be made of the following material:

- Soft nylon that snaps behind the ears (These are collapsible and easily washed.)
- Stiff leather with straps that hook into premade holes
- A combination of leather or plastic sides with straps that hook behind the head and a metal or

Is It an Emergency?

plastic mesh center (Called a cage muzzle, the advantage of this type of muzzle is that the animal can easily breathe through it and vomit if necessary.)

- Muzzles specifically designed for short-nosed dogs

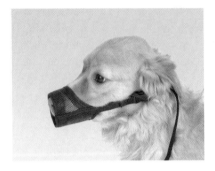

If necessary, you can fashion a homemade muzzle for most dogs, except those with very short noses (such as pugs or boxers), by following these steps:

1. Start with a piece of material at least 18 inches long. Gauze works best, but you can also use a stocking, necktie, sock, soft rope or piece of cloth.
2. Place a knot in the middle of the material to serve as an anchor.
3. Make a loop large enough to drop over the dog's nose, keeping enough distance between you and the dog's mouth so he cannot turn around and bite you. Slip the loop over the dog's nose from above and behind his head. Always allow him to know where you are at all times.

4. Tighten the loop down on top of the nose, but not so tight that you interfere with his breathing.
5. Pull an end of the material down each side of the face, crisscross it under the chin and bring the ends back behind the ears.
6. Tie the loose ends in a bow behind the ears.

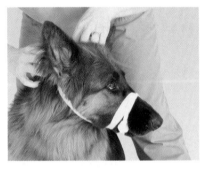

For short-nosed dogs, after steps 1–5, take one end of the material and pass it under the loop over the nose and tie it to the other end around the neck.

All hurt, sick or scared animals may be inclined to bite, so they should be muzzled before any care is attempted. But in some situations, muzzling may be dangerous to the animal; this danger must be weighed against the risk of human injury. It may be dangerous to muzzle an animal who is—

- Having difficulty breathing.
- Coughing.
- Vomiting.

NOTE: No muzzle is fool-proof, so don't be lulled into a false sense of security while using one. Many dogs can get out of a muzzle, especially if it is not fitted correctly or tied snugly.

Some animals will resist being muzzled and might become aggressive. In this case, do not attempt to muzzle the dog or care for him yourself. Take the animal to your veterinarian or seek help from your local animal shelter or animal care and control agency.

Restraint Techniques

The first two restraining techniques require two people—one to hold the dog, while the other cares for the dog. None of these techniques should be attempted unless the dog is muzzled.

Getting a Dog in a Headlock.

1. Place your forearm under the dog's neck and wrap your arm around his head.
2. Face toward the dog's back.
3. Firmly lock your forearm under the dog's head.
4. Place your other arm over or under his belly.

This position will prevent a large, powerful dog from turning around to bite, but he might still be able to overpower you.

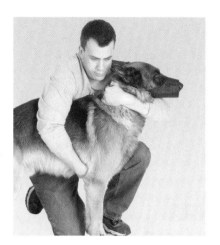

Be particularly careful with small dogs with pushed-in noses, such as pugs; holding the neck too tightly can cause the eyes to pop out of their sockets.

Laying a Dog on His Side.

1. Stand alongside and face the standing dog. **(Step 1)**

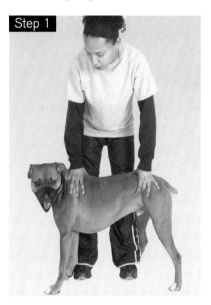

Step 1

Is It an Emergency?

2. Reach over the dog to take hold of the front and hind legs closest to your body. **(Step 2)**
3. Gently pull the legs forward. As the dog drops to the floor, be careful to prevent his head from hitting the floor.
4. Use your legs to cushion the fall.
5. Hold the front and hind legs that touch the floor straight out. **(Step 5)**

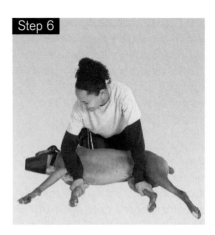

Step 6

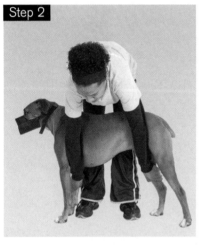

Step 2

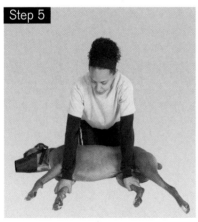

Step 5

6. Firmly push the dog's neck down against the surface on which you are working by using your forearm closest to the dog. Holding the legs straight and pushing the neck down will prevent him from standing. **(Step 6)**

If You Are Alone.
1. Place a muzzle on your dog.
2. Put a leash on your dog, and use it to restrain her head.
3. Treat the affected area.

Carrying and Transporting Techniques
If you suspect a back injury, see Broken Back or Neck, page 59, for the proper transport technique. You may also need to refer to Restraint Techniques, page 31.

Small Dog (less than 30 pounds). Carry the dog in a box or carrier if available. Follow the instructions that follow if you must carry the dog in your arms.

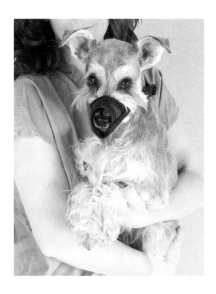

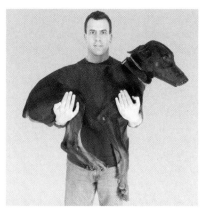

1. Cradle the dog in your arm.
2. Place your hand around the dog's front legs, with two or three fingers between her front paws.
3. Support the hind legs with your other hand.
4. Keep the injured side against your body.

Medium or Large Dog (30 pounds or greater).

1. Place one arm under and around his neck.
2. If you suspect abdominal injury, cup your other arm behind his hind legs.
3. If you suspect hind-leg injury, cup your other arm under his belly.
4. If you suspect back or neck injury, see Broken Back or Neck, page 59.

Be Prepared for Shock

Shock is the body's response to a change in blood flow and oxygen to the internal organs and tissues. It is always an emergency. It can result from a sudden loss of blood, a traumatic injury, heart failure, severe allergic reaction (anaphylactic shock), organ disease or an infection circulating through the body (septic shock). There are three stages of shock that may look very different:

- **Early shock** is when the body attempts to compensate for the decreased flow of fluids and oxygen to the tissues.
- **Middle shock** is when the body has difficulty compensating for the lack of blood flow and oxygen.
- **End stage shock** is when the body can no longer compensate for the lack of oxygen and blood flow to vital organs. This often leads to death.

See Shock, page 102, to learn how to respond to shock.

Is It an Emergency?

Emergency Conditions

The following conditions are medical emergencies requiring immediate response:

- Birthing problems
- Bleeding that is prolonged or severe, such as spurting blood, or that you cannot stop by applying direct pressure
- Breathing difficulty
- Burns
- Cuts and gashes that expose internal organs or wounds with visible bone or severe tissue damage
- Drop in body temperature (hypothermia)
- Enlarged painful abdomen
- Heat stroke (hyperthermia)
- Paralysis
- Poisoning
- Profuse diarrhea or vomiting
- Seizures, particularly first seizures, seizures lasting longer than 2 minutes and repeating seizures (repeating one after the other)
- Severe depression (characterized by hiding, unresponsiveness or refusing to eat)
- Shock
- Snake bites
- Straining to urinate or defecate
- Trauma, such as being struck by a car, shot by a gun or falling from a significant height
- Unconsciousness

Call your veterinarian or a veterinary emergency hospital immediately if your dog is affected by any of these conditions.

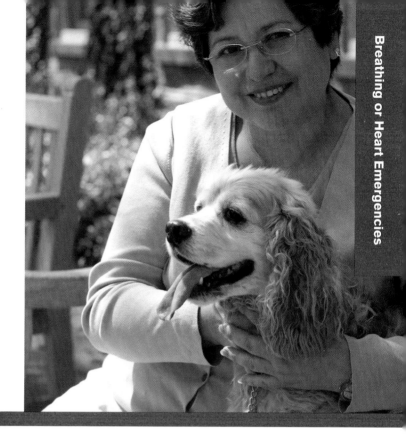

5

Respond to a Breathing or Heart Emergency

Breathing and heart problems are life-threatening emergencies. When seconds count, you won't have time to look up information so it's crucial to know how to respond before such an emergency occurs. Read this chapter carefully and watch the related segments on the DVD. This also is a good time to reflect on how well prepared you are to help your human loved ones in a similar emergency. Contact your local Red Cross chapter today and sign up for a CPR certification course. Your peace of mind is well worth this small investment of time.

Veterinary Emergency Numbers

You should know the veterinarian's emergency numbers and where the closest 24-hour emergency animal hospital is so you won't get lost trying to get there when time is critical.

Cardiopulmonary Resuscitation

Cardiopulmonary resuscitation (CPR) is used to treat an animal that is not breathing and has no heartbeat or pulse. It consists of rescue breaths (also called mouth-to-nose or mouth-to-mouth breathing) and chest compressions. CPR is based on three basic principles, called the ABCs of CPR. Follow the A-B-C order (Airway, Breathing and Circulation) when attempting CPR. See the Dog CPR Chart, page 40, for information on breathing and compression rates.

NOTE: Do not assume there is no heartbeat or pulse simply because an animal is not breathing. Do not start chest compressions before checking for a heartbeat. (If the animal is conscious and responds to you, then the heart is beating.)

Airway

The airway is the breathing passage. To open the airway and check the throat and mouth for foreign objects, take the following steps:

1. Lay the animal down, on either side.
2. Gently tilt the head slightly back to extend the neck and head.
3. Pull the tongue between the front teeth.
4. If the dog is unconscious, use your finger to check for and remove any foreign material or vomit from the mouth.

IMPORTANT: Do not place your fingers inside the mouth of a conscious animal–you may be bitten!

Breathing

After opening the airway, check to see if the dog is breathing. If not—

1. For small dogs (less than 30 pounds) and puppies, cover and seal the dog's entire snout with your mouth and exhale until you see the chest rise. **(Step 1A)** For medium, large and giant dogs (30 pounds or more), gently hold the muzzle closed. Place

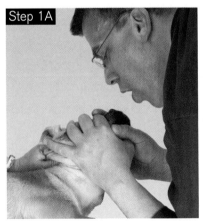
Step 1A

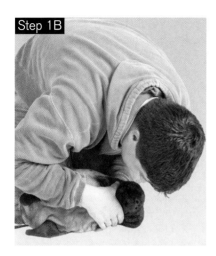

Step 1B

your mouth over the dog's nose and gently exhale until you see the chest rise. **(Step 1B)**

2. Give 4 or 5 breaths rapidly, then check to see if your pet is breathing without assistance. If he begins to breathe, but the breathing is shallow and irregular or if breathing does not begin, continue giving him rescue breaths until you reach the veterinary hospital or for up to 20 minutes. Beyond 20 minutes there is little chance of reviving your pet. (See Breathing Rate on the Dog CPR Chart, page 40.)

NOTE: Do not attempt this on a conscious animal!

Circulation

Is there a heartbeat or a pulse? If not, perform chest compressions. (See Heart Rate and Pulse, Compression Position and Compression Rate on the Dog CPR Chart, page 40.)

Here is how to best position various-sized dogs for CPR:

Small Dog (less than 30 pounds).

1. With the dog lying down on her right side, kneel with her chest facing you.
2. Place the palm of one hand over her ribs at the point where her elbow touches the chest, just behind the front legs.
3. Place your other hand underneath her right side. **(Step 3)**
4. Compress the chest ½ to 1 inch or by 25–35 percent of her chest width (your elbows should be softly locked during compressions).

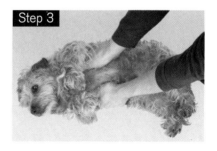

Step 3

Medium to Large Dog (30–90 pounds).

1. Have the dog lie down on his right side.
2. If you are alone, have the dog's chest facing you. If there are two people, you should stand or kneel with the dog's back toward you, while the other person gives rescue breaths.

3. Extend your arms at the elbows.
4. Cup your hands over each other.
5. Compress the chest at the point where the left elbow lies when pulled back to the chest or at the widest part of the rib cage. **(Step 5)**
6. Compress the chest about 1–3 inches (25–35 percent of the chest width) with each compression.

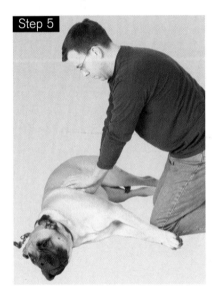

Step 5

Giant Dogs (more than 90 pounds). Use the same chest compression technique as for medium to large dogs.

Choking

Dogs can choke on food or toys in an instant. But you can help by following the suggestions below.

Signs and Symptoms.
- Anxiousness, dog acts frantic
- Dog stops breathing
- Gums may be blue or white
- Loud breathing sounds
- Pawing at the mouth
- Struggling or gasping to breathe

The Most Common Causes.
- Ill animal choking on its own vomit
- Object stuck in throat
- Tongue swelling due to an allergic reaction
- Trauma to neck or throat region
- Upper respiratory disease

What You Can Do. Use caution to avoid being bitten, especially if working on a conscious or semi-conscious animal.

Open the mouth and carefully sweep the inside with your finger to try to feel and dislodge the object. Be careful not to push the object farther into the throat.

1. Pull the tongue forward, removing any object, vomit or foreign material present. (See Airway, page 36.)
2. Perform abdominal thrusts by either lifting up the dog, standing behind or next to the dog, or laying the dog down. For dogs that can be lifted, lift the dog by the front legs with the spine against your chest and wrap your arms around the animal under the ribs, or if standing behind the dog, bend over and wrap your arms around the animal under the ribs. Make a

fist with one hand, place your other hand over your fist and give 5 rapid abdominal thrusts, lifting your fist in an inward and upward motion. **(Step 2)** If the dog is too heavy to lift, place the dog on her side, place the head and neck in a neutral position, place the palms of your hand below the rib cage and give 5 rapid abdominal thrusts in a inward and upward motion.

3. Check the animal's mouth with a penlight to see if the object is dislodged.

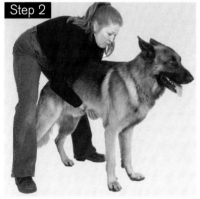

Step 2

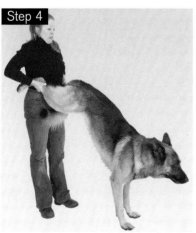

Step 4

4. If this is unsuccessful, and the dog can be lifted, suspend the animal by the hips with the head hanging down. If the animal is too large to suspend, hold the animal's hind legs in the air (like a wheelbarrow) so the head hangs down. **(Step 4)**

5. Next check the animal's mouth; remove the object if possible.

6. If you cannot dislodge the object, give 5 sharp back blows between the shoulder blades using the palm of your hand. **(Step 6)**

7. Carefully sweep the dog's mouth with your finger to dislodge the object, if it has not already come out on its own.

8. If the dog becomes unconscious, give 5 rescue breaths (see Breathing, page 36) and give 5 quick abdominal thrusts, then check the mouth again.

9. Once the object is dislodged, stop abdominal thrusts, check the dog's ABCs, and begin CPR if needed. (See CPR, page 36.)

10. Take the dog to a veterinary hospital at once.

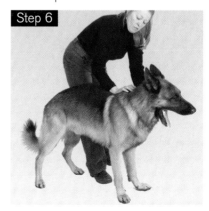

Step 6

DOG CPR CHART

	Small (Less than 30 pounds)	Medium or Large (30 to 90 pounds)	Giant (More than 90 pounds)
Breaths-to-Compressions Ratio	• 1 breath then 5 compressions with 1 rescuer • 1 breath then 3 compressions with 2 rescuers	• 1 breath then 5 compressions with 1 rescuer • 1 breath then 3 compressions with 2 rescuers	• 1 breath then 10 compressions with 1 rescuer • 1 breath then 6 compressions with 2 rescuers
Breathing Position	• Cover and seal dog's mouth and nose with your mouth and exhale until you see the chest rise.	• Gently hold muzzle closed. Place your mouth over animal's nose and exhale until you see the chest rise.	
Breathing Rate	• 20 to 30 breaths per minute	• 20 breaths per minute	
Compression Position	• With dog's chest facing you, place one hand over and the other hand under his ribs, just behind the front legs. • Squeeze your hands together. • Compress the chest about ½ to 1 inch each time.	• If one rescuer, have the dog's chest facing you. If two rescuers, one person should stand or kneel with the dog's back toward him or her, while the other person will provide rescue breaths. • Extend your arms at the elbows. • Cup one hand over the other. • Compress the chest either at the widest part of the chest OR at the point where the dog's left elbow lies when pulled back to the chest. • Compress the chest about 1 to 3 inches each time.	
Compression Rate	• 100 to 120 chest compressions per minute—about 2–3 per second	• 100 chest compressions per minute—about 2 per second	
How Long Should You Perform CPR?	• Perform cycles of rescue breaths and chest compressions (CPR), then check for a pulse or breathing every 2-3 minutes. • If no pulse, continue CPR until the animal has a strong heartbeat and pulse, until you reach the veterinary hospital, or until 20 minutes have passed and your efforts have not been successful.		

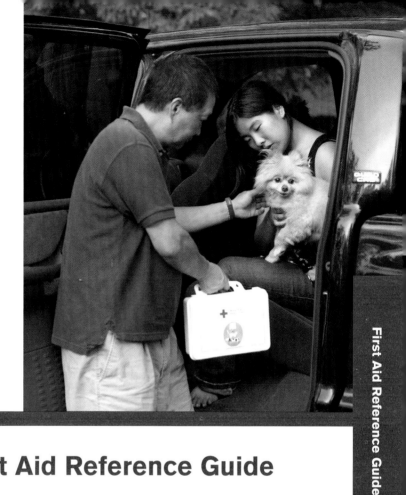

6

First Aid Reference Guide

If you turned to this section of the book because you are worried about your sick or injured dog, remain calm. Look for your pet's condition or symptoms in this section of the book; the topics are arranged alphabetically. Many subject areas will refer you to other topics where you will find even more information to help your dog, as well as help you determine if you need to take him to a veterinarian.

Abrasions

Abrasions—scrapes to the skin's top layers—can be shallow and heal easily or large and more serious. Your dog may lick or scratch the area, which may appear red or ooze blood.

What You Can Do.
1. Wash your hands and put on nonlatex, disposable gloves.
2. Apply a sterile, water-soluble (not petroleum-based) lubricant (see Pet First Aid Kit, page 18) so hair does not contaminate the wound while you shave the area.
3. Clip hair around the area gently with grooming clippers or, as a last resort, scissors. If using scissors, do not cut too close to the skin and be sure to keep the scissors parallel so that you'll be less likely to poke the skin if your dog moves suddenly.
4. Flush the wound with warm water or saline solution (add 1 teaspoon of salt to 1 quart of warm water to make solution) to remove the skin lubricant.
5. Then wash the wound with water or saline solution to remove any remaining dirt or debris. If necessary, wet a gauze sponge with sterile saline solution to clean any remaining debris.

Take your dog to the veterinarian if the abrasion is larger than a quarter, seems painful, is red, does not begin to heal after 2–3 days, oozes a yellow or foul-smelling discharge or if you are unsure of its depth or severity.

Allergies and Allergic Reactions
Insect Bites

During warm weather, dogs are susceptible to spider bites and bee stings. Insects often sting the soft, less hairy areas of your pet, such as the nose and feet. These sometimes cause allergic reactions.

Signs and Symptoms.
- Collapse (See Collapse, page 63.)
- Difficulty breathing
- Pain, itching, licking at the site
- Redness, discoloration or hives (bumps in the skin) around the site, sometimes spreading to other body parts
- Red bumps on the abdomen, vomiting or diarrhea and swelling at the sting site, which may spread and include the face, especially around the eyes, and neck

NOTE: A severe allergic reaction can lead to anaphylactic shock. This could occur immediately or progressively over several hours. (See Shock, page 102.)

What You Can Do.
1. If your dog's face and neck are swollen, check his airway, breathing and circulation (ABCs). (See Airway, Breathing and Circulation, pages 36–37.) If your dog cannot breathe, begin rescue breathing. (See Cardiopulmonary Resuscitation, page 36.) If your dog's breathing is noisy or labored, take him to a veterinarian immediately.

2. Check for signs of shock. (See Shock, page 102.)
3. Check if the stinger is still present; it's usually black and very small. Do not attempt to pick it out, as this may release more toxin. Instead, scrape it off with a firm object, such as your fingernail or a credit card.
4. Apply cold compress or ice packs wrapped in a towel to help control swelling.
5. Transport your dog to a veterinary hospital. (See How to Approach, Capture and Restrain a Dog, page 28.)
6. It may be appropriate to give your dog the over-the-counter antihistamine diphenhydramine (Benadryl®), **if your veterinarian has given approval.** Many over-the-counter products contain diphenhydramine along with other cold or allergy medications (i.e., acetaminophen or pseudoephedrine). **It is extremely important to ensure that the**

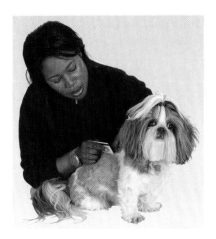

product contains diphenhydramine ONLY.

Diphenhydramine (Benedryl®) Dosing. In general, the dose is 2 mg per dog's weight in kg. You can convert your dog's weight by the equation: 1 kg = 2.2 pounds.

- Small dogs (less than 30 pounds): 10 mg
- Medium dogs (30 to 50 pounds): 25 mg
- Large and giant dogs (greater than 50 pounds): 50 mg

Give oral medication only if your dog is conscious, able to breathe and not vomiting!

Skin Allergies
Allergies are one of the most common causes of skin conditions in dogs.

Signs and Symptoms. Itchiness, swelling, red skin or red bumps, with or without a white center— pustules and papules, most common on the lower abdomen (belly)

The Most Common Causes. Flea bites, food, flea and tick products, grass, mold, pollen and other plants, grooming products and household cleaning products

What You Can Do.
1. Wash your dog thoroughly using a very mild soap or baby shampoo.
2. Apply a compress, such as a cold, wet washcloth, to the affected area.

First Aid Reference Guide

3. Administer diphenhydramine (Benadryl®), if approved by your veterinarian.
4. Talk to your veterinarian about potential causes and treatment (i.e., food elimination trial). A secondary infection may develop, requiring oral antibiotics.

Anal Sac Swelling/ Infection/Abscess

If you notice your dog frequently licking at or scooting his hind quarters around the house or yard it might be because he's trying to express an impacted anal gland that's making him uncomfortable. Dogs usually express these glands upon defecating. An impacted anal gland is not only painful, but it can become infected and abscessed.

Signs and Symptoms. Anorexia, fever, lethargy, redness, pressure, pain, licking at and scooting the area, possibly discharge/pus on one side of the anus

What You Can Do. Take your dog to the veterinarian. If the gland is impacted, a veterinarian can express it. If it's infected or abscessed, the veterinarian will sedate your dog to lance and flush the swelling, then give oral antibiotics.

Prevention. Always have your veterinarian check anal glands during checkups; if your dog is prone to scooting and impacted anal glands, your veterinarian can teach you

how to express these glands at home to keep them empty.

Balance, Loss of (Vestibular Disease)

Vestibular disease causes a dog to lose his balance. It can strike a dog at any age, but older dogs are more at risk. It isn't always life threatening—even though it mimics a stroke. However, it is serious and needs immediate attention. Many dogs with a less serious case compensate well and overcome it.

The Most Common Causes. Brain disease, foreign object in the ear, inner ear infection, parasitic disease and a problem with the balance center in the brain (called idiopathic peripheral vestibular disease)

Signs and Symptoms. Change in behavior, circling in one direction, drooling, eyes appearing to move rapidly from side to side or up and down, falling to one side, head tilting to one side and vomiting

What You Can Do.
1. Any animal with these symptoms should be examined by a veterinarian as soon as possible.
2. Look inside your dog's ears. If they are red, swollen or contain a lot of debris, he may have an ear infection. Take him to a veterinarian for treatment. Prolonged, untreated ear infections can lead to hearing loss or brain infections.

If the veterinarian diagnoses peripheral vestibular disease, it is crucial to keep your dog out of danger and away from staircases, balconies and open windows. And don't allow him free reign outdoors. It is not known what causes idiopathic peripheral vestibular disease, but it tends to occur in the warmer months and is more common in older dogs. The good news is that peripheral vestibular disease generally clears up on its own, in about 2–6 weeks. However, your dog must be examined by a veterinarian to rule out more serious brain diseases, including central vestibular disease.

Birthing Emergencies (Dystocia)

In a perfect world, every dog would have a home. Unfortunately, we don't live in a perfect world. Spaying or neutering your dog is crucial to control pet overpopulation (and dog homelessness), and it also has positive health and behavioral benefits. (See Spaying and Neutering, page 5.) But sometimes the unexpected happens. You may take in a stray or otherwise acquire a pregnant dog. If you suspect pregnancy, take the dog to your veterinarian for advice and treatment. Once you know she's pregnant, prepare in advance by providing a whelping box, bedding and a heat source. If you are faced with an unexpected birth, use the following information as a guide.

In dogs, normal pregnancies last 62–64 days. About a day before giving birth, the dog's body temperature decreases to less than 100° F, she may have a decreased appetite and her nesting behavior (gathering materials for a bed) may get very intense.

Labor and Delivery

Stage one—the cervix dilates. The dog generally appears nervous or anxious and may pace, pant and lie down and get up a lot; this may last for 12–24 hours. Contractions will not be visible.

Stage two—forceful visible uterine contractions occur. She actively strains to expel each puppy. These contractions look as if she is trying to defecate while lying on her side, and she probably will pant. Stage two labor usually lasts from 3–6 hours, but it may last up to 10–12 hours or more if she is disturbed or is having a large litter. If the contractions are weak, a puppy could be born every 3–4 hours, but if contractions are strong and forceful the puppies could be born about 30 minutes apart. The first puppy should be born within 1–2 hours after stage two labor begins.

Stage three—the placenta should come out with each puppy or shortly afterward. The whole process should last between 3 and 24 hours.

Normal Position of Puppies.

Slightly more than half of puppies are born head first, and the rest are born rear-end first. Both presentations are normal.

After Birth. The mother should clean off each puppy after it is born and sever the umbilical cord with her teeth. Usually, she will eat the placenta. The mother will have a red, brown or dark-green vaginal discharge (lochia), which may persist for up to 6 weeks, but should become less profuse after the first few days. Take her to a veterinarian if this discharge appears bright red, contains pus or has a foul odor, as these are signs of infection.

Birthing Problems
The Most Common Causes.
- Deformed or dead fetus
- The mother's pelvis is too small, the puppy is too large or the mother had a prior pelvic injury, such as a fracture
- Weak uterine contractions or twisted uterus

Signs and Symptoms.
- More than 2 days past the dog's due date or past a temperature drop (if known) or a dark vaginal discharge with a foul odor
- Active labor for more than 4 hours with no puppy
- More than 30 minutes of active continuous straining between puppies with no puppy produced (Active straining is an obvious contraction with the dog trying to push.)
- Puppy at the vulva, but mother unable to push it out within 20 minutes
- Mother looking weak, sick and depressed
- Mother biting or whining at vulva area
- Bloody discharge before birth

It is a good idea to check on your dog, but do not be overly attentive. If the dog is in active labor for 4 or more hours with no puppy, or if more than 2 hours pass between puppies, or she has any of the above signs, call a veterinarian *immediately* for an assessment, and be prepared to get her to a veterinary hospital. At the veterinary hospital, the attending doctor may attempt to treat her with medication to increase the force of contractions. Otherwise, a cesarean section may be performed.

Note: Some dogs will stop labor if they are disturbed.

What You Can Do. If the puppy is visible but the mother cannot push any longer—

1. Put on nonlatex, disposable gloves (preferably sterile).
2. Gently grasp the puppy with a clean towel.
3. When the mother bears down (during an active contraction) help pull the puppy gently out of the vulva toward you in a slightly downward direction. **Do not pull the puppy when the mother is not pushing.** You can easily dislocate or fracture bones if the fetus is pulled too vigorously.

If the mother is not cleaning up the puppy—

1. Allow the mother to try to clean the puppy. If she doesn't, remove the puppy from the sac and

clean the mouth, nose (to remove any fluid) and eyes with a clean cloth.
2. Rub gently (but vigorously) to stimulate breathing.
3. Dry the puppy with a cloth. Cut the umbilical cord, but only after the puppy is breathing and its gums are pink.

To cut the cord properly—

1. Tie a piece of fishing line, dental floss or heavy string snugly around the cord about 1 inch from the body.
2. Make a second tie about ½ inch from the first. (Do not pull on the cord as this can cause a hernia.)
3. Cut between the two ties.

If the puppy is not breathing—

1. Wipe the puppy with a towel. Clear the face, nose, eyes and mouth.
2. Hold the puppy firmly in your hand with the head pointing down.
3. Clean away fluid from the nose and mouth. (You can suction gently with a baby dosing syringe or bulb syringe.)
4. If the newborn is still not breathing, perform rescue breathing. (See CPR, page 36.) You do not have to seal off the mouth when performing rescue breathing because the newborn should be small enough for you to put your mouth over both the puppy's mouth and nose.

5. Repeat vigorous wiping with a towel, holding the puppy on a slight downward slant to drain any fluids. Continue to perform rescue breathing as needed. (See CPR, page 36.) Do not shake or jostle the newborn.

If you suspect a problem, call your veterinarian immediately!

Bite Wounds

It's scary to see your dog engaged in a dogfight, and it can be extremely dangerous. Never try to break up a dogfight yourself—you could be bitten.

Bite wounds can look minor but be deep and serious, so if your dog is bitten by a dog or other animal, take him to a veterinarian as soon as possible to prevent the wound from becoming infected.

Signs and Symptoms. Small wound in skin, most likely two puncture marks; bleeding; bruising, particularly if a larger attacking dog picks up and shakes a smaller dog, which also can cause significant internal injuries

If a wound is not immediately apparent, the injured dog may develop an infection or abscess 1 or 2 days after being bitten.

Signs of bite wound infection include: fever, usually above 103° F; lethargy; loss of appetite; pain when affected area is touched.

First Aid Reference Guide

First Aid Reference Guide   47

An **abscess** is a soft swelling around the wound. If unruptured, the top of the swelling may be red or blue, painful and look taut. If ruptured, pus will be visible, often accompanied by a foul odor.

If your dog has an abscess that has not ruptured, take your dog to a veterinarian as soon as possible for abscess care. If the abscess has ruptured, clean the area as described under Abrasions, page 42, and take him to a veterinarian.

What You Can Do.
1. If the wound is bleeding excessively, control the bleeding. (See Bleeding, page 48.)
2. Check the dog's ABCs; perform CPR as needed. (See CPR, page 36.)
3. Check for shock. (See Shock, page 102.)
4. Administer basic wound care. (See Abrasions, page 42.)

If you witness the bite, find out the rabies vaccination status of the attacking dog. Recheck the rabies vaccination status of the bitten dog. If your pet was bitten by a wild animal and the wild animal is dead, take it to the veterinarian so it can be sent to a laboratory for a rabies examination.

Note: Wear nonlatex, disposable gloves, place the animal in a plastic bag, then seal the bag. Do not attempt to capture a live wild animal.

If you suspect a snakebite, see Venomous Bites and Stings (Snakes, Scorpions, Toads and Jellyfish), page 109.

Bleeding
There are two types of serious bleeding. Arterial bleeding, characterized by rhythmically spurting blood, is more rapid and profuse and therefore more difficult to stop. Venal bleeding is slower and less profuse. It is much easier to stop and less dangerous.

(For nosebleeds, see Nosebleeds, page 89. For bleeding ear flaps, see Ear Problems, page 69.)

What You Can Do.
1. Wearing nonlatex, disposable gloves, hold a piece of gauze, wash cloth or other clean material over the bleeding site and apply direct pressure. **(Step 1)** If the material becomes soaked through, do not remove it but apply another cloth over it. Do this repeatedly if necessary. Direct pressure is the safest way

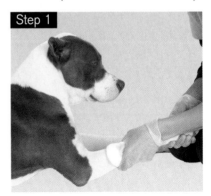
Step 1

to stop bleeding until you can reach a veterinary hospital.

2. If bleeding has not stopped and blood is spurting, in addition to direct pressure over the wound, hold the area just *above* the wound with your hand in an effort to close off the blood vessel. If blood is flowing heavily but not spurting, hold the area just *below* the bleeding site to close off the blood vessels.

3. If this fails to stop the bleeding, apply a pressure bandage.
   • Wrap gauze or other soft material around the wound just tight enough to stop the bleeding. Do not make it too tight. **(Step 3A)**
   • Secure with tape. **(Step 3B)**
   • If you wrapped a limb, check repeatedly for swelling of the toes or toes that become cold; these indicate your bandage is too tight, in which case you will need to loosen it.

4. If the limb does not appear to be broken, elevate the limb above the heart, while continuing to apply direct pressure.

5. If none of the above techniques work, apply hand pressure to pressure points (see below).

6. Take your dog to a veterinarian immediately.

Pressure Point Technique

To use the pressure point technique, apply firm, even pressure to the appropriate pressure point:

• ***Bleeding on the front limbs.*** Press three fingers up and into the armpit on the side with the bleeding limb.

• ***Bleeding on the back limbs.*** Press three fingers on the area of the inner thigh where the leg meets the body wall on the side with the bleeding limb.

• ***Bleeding of the head.*** Press three fingers at the base of the lower jaw (the angle just below the ear) on the same side and below where the bleeding is occurring.

First Aid Reference Guide

Step 3A

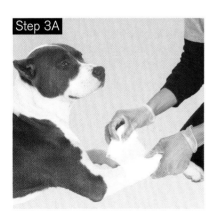

Step 3B

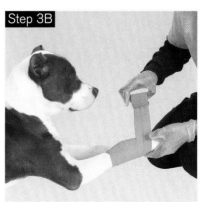

- ***Bleeding of the neck.*** Press three fingers in the soft groove next to the windpipe (which feels round and hard) just below the wound on the side of the neck where the bleeding is occurring. Be sure to *not* apply pressure to the windpipe itself.

When using pressure points to control bleeding, you must release pressure slightly, for a few seconds, at least every 10 minutes. This helps prevent permanent damage.

IMPORTANT: Avoid using the neck pressure point on any animal suspected of having a head injury, unless you feel the animal's life is in immediate danger. Be sure you do not restrict breathing.

Tourniquet Technique
Use only on the limbs—never place a tourniquet around the neck!

1. Wrap a strip of cloth or gauze (about 2 inches wide) twice around the limb above the bleeding area. **DO NOT MAKE A KNOT.**
2. Tighten the gauze or cloth by wrapping each end around a rigid object, such as a stick.
3. Turn the stick slowly and just enough to stop blood flow. Write the time on a piece of tape on the tourniquet.
4. Loosen the tie for several seconds at least every 10 minutes to help avoid permanent tissue damage.

5. Be aware that the interrupted blood supply may cause your dog to lose the limb.
6. Take your dog to a veterinarian immediately.

NOTE: Pressure points and tourniquets should be used only as a last resort, in a life-or-death situation. (For example, the animal has lost enough blood to lose consciousness.) Persistent decreased blood flow to the area may cause severe damage.

Bloat and Torsion
Bloat and torsion are life-threatening conditions that are more common in deep-chested large and giant dogs. Gastric dilation, or bloat, is when the dog's stomach overfills with air or food. Torsion, or volvulus, is a worsening of this condition in which the stomach turns around upon itself, often misplacing the spleen with it. This cuts off the blood supply to both organs and prevents blood from returning to the heart. **Know the signs of bloat so you can save your dog's life by getting her to the veterinarian sooner.**

Signs and Symptoms. The signs of bloat often occur within hours after a meal. These include: drooling or salivation; distended abdomen (enlargement of the stomach area); non-productive retching or vomiting; restlessness and pacing; and shock.

The Most Common Causes. Bloat and torsion are thought to be associated with eating large meals, exercising just before or after eating and gorging on large amounts of food or water. However, the exact cause is unknown.

What You Can Do.
1. Check the dog's ABCs; perform CPR as needed. (See CPR, page 36.)
2. Check for signs of shock. (See Shock, page 102.)
3. **Take her to a veterinary hospital immediately.**

Your dog must have anti-shock fluid therapy, be assessed for stomach rotation (with an x-ray) and have her stomach decompressed. **Once your dog is stable, emergency surgery will be necessary for a rotated stomach.**

Prevention. Although there are no foolproof ways to prevent bloat, some things may help:

* Feed your dog more than once daily. Two meals of equal size are best.
* Do not allow your dog to exercise immediately before or after a meal; wait at least 1 hour.
* Do not give your dog access to bulk food sources from which she might gorge herself.
* Do not allow your dog to drink a large volume of water at one time, particularly immediately after exercise or eating.

Blood Calcium, Low, Eclampsia (Following Birth)

Eclampsia, or low blood calcium, may occur in female dogs during late pregnancy and up to 2–4 weeks after giving birth. It is most common in small breeds. The condition can be life threatening because the lactating dog cannot meet the increasing demands of blood calcium or move calcium into her milk supply without depleting it in her own blood. Low blood calcium can also be caused by an endocrine disease (hypoparathyroidism).

Calcium is needed for muscle activity, so muscle tremors and seizures can occur when the blood calcium level drops sharply.

Signs and Symptoms. Muscle tremors, which may involve the whole body; seizures; fever; restlessness; nervousness; stiff gait or inability to walk

What You Can Do.
1. **Take your pet to a veterinary hospital immediately.**
2. Puppies should stop nursing and be given a supplemental formula. Ask your veterinarian for instructions on how to do this.

Prevention. Feed a pregnant dog puppy food 2–3 weeks before delivery and continue for 4 weeks after delivery. Have your dog spayed.

Blood in Urine

Red-colored urine signals the presence of blood and is probably due to a urinary tract infection. Antibiotics will most likely clear it up. But it could indicate a bladder stone, tumor or even poisoning. So it's important to get your dog to a veterinarian as soon as possible to determine the cause.

The Most Common Causes.

Bladder infection, usually bacterial, less commonly fungal or parasitic; bleeding disorder; heat cycle (estrus in a female); inflammation, due to stones or crystals in the bladder; kidney infection; poisoning (rat poison); prostate disease; trauma; tumor or uterine infection in a female

What You Can Do.

1. Watch carefully to be sure your pet is able to pass or produce urine.
2. Check for other signs, such as vomiting, not eating or lethargy.
3. In the case of a nonspayed female, look at her vulva to see if there is a discharge. A small amount of blood-tinged urine is normal for a dog in heat, but if the discharge contains pus and smells foul, she may have a uterine infection known as a pyometra. (See Vaginal Discharge and Uterine Infection, page 108.)
4. Take your dog to a veterinarian. If possible, bring a new, clean urine specimen from the animal. Catch a specimen by placing a clean shallow cup, such as a margarine tub or aluminum foil pie plate, in the urine stream. It is best to obtain the specimen the same day you go to the veterinarian, but if this is not possible, you can place the specimen in the refrigerator overnight. If you cannot obtain your dog's urine specimen at home, then prevent your dog from urinating outside for at least 1 hour prior to the veterinary visit so the veterinarian can get a sample.

Prevention. Neuter your male dog to reduce the risk of prostate disease (infection and enlargement). Spay your female dog to prevent uterine infections.

If your dog is being treated for a urinary tract infection, administering your pet's antibiotics as prescribed can help prevent future infections. Also, adhere to any special diet or other medication your veterinarian prescribes.

Blood in Stool

Signs and Symptoms. Bright red blood in or on top of stool or—more serious—melena, a black, tarry stool

The Most Common Causes.

Colitis; straining while defecating; stomach ulcer causing bleeding in the upper intestines

What You Can Do. Call the veterinarian immediately whenever you observe blood in your dog's stool.

Blood Sugar Emergencies

Blood sugar emergencies can be life threatening and are often caused by diabetes. They can occur abruptly if the blood sugar level is too high (hyperglycemia) or too low (hypoglycemia). It's important to monitor your pet's glucose level (usually in urine) if he is diabetic. Most diabetic dogs require insulin injections once or twice daily, although some may be regulated through oral medications or diet alone.

Hyperglycemia

Hyperglycemia is when the blood sugar level is too high. One of the most common causes of hyperglycemia is *diabetes mellitus*, which is the abnormal metabolism of insulin. If a diabetic dog's blood sugar is too high and he develops another health problem, he can go into a diabetic ketoacidotic state. This is a life-threatening emergency.

Signs and Symptoms. Increased appetite, increased thirst, increased urination, and weight loss

If your dog has diabetes and progresses to a diabetic ketoacidosis state, secondary disease processes can occur including—

• Change in behavior
• Dehydration (See Dehydration, page 65.)
• Increased breathing rate
• Loss of appetite
• Shock and death if untreated
• Sweet smell to breath (ketones)
• Weakness
• Vomiting

Causes of Hyperglycemia Due to Diabetes Mellitus. Inadequate insulin regulation, undiagnosed diabetes mellitus, incorrect insulin dose, increased insulin demand, insulin not properly administered

Causes of Hyperglycemia Not Due to Diabetes Mellitus. Dog gorges on a bulk food source, glandular or endocrine disease, organ disease or stress

What You Can Do.
1. Check the dog's ABCs; perform CPR as needed. (See CPR, page 36.)
2. Check for shock. (See Shock, page 102.)
3. Take your dog to a veterinary hospital as soon as possible. Be sure to take his insulin and syringe with you.

Hypoglycemia

Hypoglycemia occurs when the blood sugar level is too low. The most common cause is insulin overdose.

Signs and Symptoms. Coma or unconsciousness; disorientation; seizures; shaking; weakness; wobbly, drunken-looking gait

First Aid Reference Guide

Causes of Hypoglycemia Due to Diabetes Mellitus or Receiving Insulin.

- Not eating after receiving an insulin injection (You should always feed your pet prior to giving him the insulin.)
- Overdose of insulin, which can be caused by the wrong insulin syringe being used, a change in the type of insulin being used or improper administration
- Reduced need for insulin
- Vomiting up a meal after receiving an insulin injection

Causes of Hypoglycemia Not Due to Diabetes Mellitus or Receiving Insulin.

- Liver disease
- Loss of appetite—mostly in young puppies
- Poor nutrition in very young animals
- Severe infection/sepsis
- Tumor that secretes insulin

What You Can Do.

1. Check the dog's ABCs; perform CPR as needed. (See CPR, page 36.)
2. Rub corn syrup on the gums, but do not force it into the mouth. Do this even if your pet is comatose. An oral glucose paste is sold at pharmacies; if you know your pet is diabetic or has a history of low blood sugar, keep this product in your first aid kit.
3. If you do not have the glucose paste or corn syrup, rub sugar water on the gums.
4. Take the animal to a veterinary hospital immediately.

Bone, Dislocated (Out of Joint)/Subluxation

The two most common joints to become luxated (completely dislocated) are the hip and elbow. Congenital disease and trauma can cause an elbow to become luxated. Hip dysplasia is the leading cause of subluxations (partial dislocation) in the hip joint, whereas trauma and hip dysplasia can cause a luxated hip joint. In any case, your dog must see a veterinarian immediately.

Signs and Symptoms.
Hip
- Animal feels pain when you feel or touch the area
- Dislocated hind leg is shorter or longer than the other
- Foot on dislocated leg does not reach the ground when the animal stands

Elbow
- Elbow is bent.
- Foot does not reach the ground.
- Lower leg is pointed away from or toward the body.
- Animal feels pain when you feel or touch the area.

What You Can Do.
1. Check the dog's ABCs; perform CPR as needed. (See CPR, page 36.)
2. Check for shock. (See Shock, page 102.)
3. In the case of the elbow, you can attempt to splint the limb in the position found (see

Fractures, below), but only if your dog cannot be immobilized and transported immediately to a veterinary hospital.

4. Transport your dog to a veterinary hospital as soon as possible. The sooner you get her to the hospital, the greater the chance the bone can be placed back in the joint without surgery.

Bone, Muscle and Joint Injuries

Dogs who don't get regular vigorous exercise are at greater risk of injuries. So, just like you, your dog should start an exercise program slowly under your watchful eye and with your veterinarian's guidance.

Sprains and Strains

A sprain is an injury involving a ligament (the tissue that connects bones to bones or bones to muscles). A strain is an injury to a muscle.

Signs and Symptoms.

- Limping (not placing the limb down at all or placing less weight on it)
- Pain when the area is touched
- Swelling

What You Can Do.

1. Apply either a cold compress (ice pack or chemical cold pack) or warm compresses to the injured area three or four times daily, for 5–15 minutes each time. Alternate warm and cold, using warm for one application, then cold for the next. Place a towel between the compresses and the skin.

2. Restrict exercise. Keep the animal in a small closed, confined area; walk on a leash only to defecate and urinate.

3. If there is no improvement in 24 hours, or if the injury worsens, seek veterinary attention. An x-ray will need to be taken to make sure there are no fractures or torn ligaments.

Never give aspirin or any other over-the-counter pain relievers to your pet unless prescribed by your veterinarian. These drugs can be very toxic to dogs!

Fractures

Fractures are breaks in the bone. They may occur singularly, in one part of the bone, or there may be multiple breaks in the bone or multiple bones involved. Fractures can have smooth, clean surfaces or have splinters and fragments.

Fractures are assessed for severity based on—

- Location of the fracture.
- Whether a joint is involved.
- Whether it is a clean break (there may be chips or splinters present).
- Whether the fracture is straight or at an angle.
- Whether the fracture site is closed or open (with bone sticking through the skin).
- Whether the growth regions of the bone are affected, in the case of young animals.

Signs and Symptoms.
- Disfigurement (part of the limb seems to be abnormally positioned)
- Lameness (not placing full weight on a limb)
- Pain
- Piece of bone sticking through the skin
- Possible bruising (which can be difficult to see under the fur)
- Swelling

What You Can Do.
1. Keep your dog as quiet and calm as possible.
2. Check the dog's ABCs; perform CPR as needed. (See CPR, page 36.)
3. If a piece of bone is protruding from the fracture site—
   - Wash the area with water or saline (add one teaspoon of salt to a quart of warm water to make solution). (The animal may not allow this.)
   - Loosely place a dressing over the wound, extending several inches past the opening. Preferably use a sterile dressing such as a nonstick pad or a gauze sponge, or use any clean piece of cloth.
   - Wrap the ends of the dressing with tape. Extend the tape several inches past the opening. Make sure you do not disturb the bones or wrap the dressing too tightly.
4. If you cannot transport your dog in a box, carrier or cage or oth-erwise keep him completely still, you can try to splint the fracture (see below).

Splinting
Splints are placed to keep the fracture immobilized to prevent further damage, and can be used for fractures at or below the elbow and at or below the knee.

To correctly immobilize a fracture, the joints on top of and below the fracture site must be included in the splint.

1. After washing and dressing the area as discussed in Step 3 (above), splint the limb in the position you find it.
2. Place a rigid structure along each side of the fractured limb. You can use rolled-up newspaper, sticks, tongue depressors or pens (for small dogs). **(Step 2)**
3. Hold the splint in place with tape placed at multiple sites surrounding the splint and limb, or with cloth strips, wrapped and tied around the limb and splint at multiple spots. **(Step 3)**
4. Do not disturb the bones—try to hold both sides of the fracture steady, and don't wrap too tightly. **(Step 4)**
5. If no rigid material is available, the uninjured leg may act as a splint. Tape or tie the uninjured leg to the injured leg, placing a thin layer of cotton or cloth between them, if possible.

6. Make sure your tape or ties are not so tight they cut off circulation. To monitor this, make sure you can always place two fingers between the tape or cloth and the limb. **(Step 6)**

For a small dog, place him in a small carrier or box. If a hip or shoulder is broken, transport your dog to a veterinary hospital immediately, keeping her as immobilized as possible on a board (or other rigid structure), box or carrier.

NOTE: Splinting a limb incorrectly can cause more damage. If you are unsure about splinting a limb or if your dog struggles too much, it is better to transport the pet in a box or carrier, or in a fashion that causes the least movement to your dog on the way to the veterinary hospital.

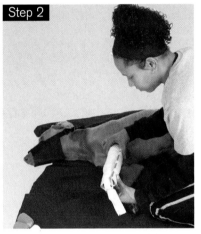

Step 2

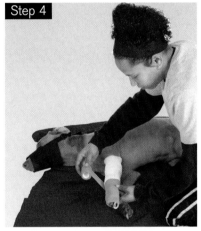

Step 4

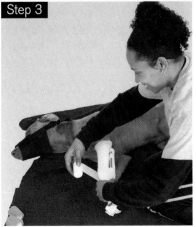

Step 3

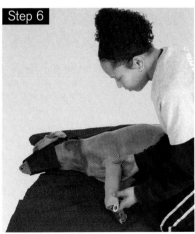

Step 6

First Aid Reference Guide

Breathing Problems

When your dog has a breathing problem, it is very important to first make sure that she's not choking. If she is, see Choking, page 62. If she's not choking but is having trouble breathing, get her to the nearest veterinary hospital immediately.

Signs and Symptoms.
- Abdomen moves when breathing
- Coughing
- Head and neck extended forward, elbows pushed out
- Increased breathing rate and effort
- Loud, noisy breathing
- Pale or blue gums (mucous membranes) (See Know What's Normal, page 24.)

The Most Common Causes.
- Lung infections such as pneumonia, which may be caused by bacteria, viruses, fungi and parasites
- Heart disease/congestive heart failure
- Upper airway disease
- Trauma (i.e., hit by a car)
- Electrical shock
- Inhaled objects or vomit
- Cancer

Upper Airway Disease or Obstruction
Brachycephalic Syndrome. This is common in breeds with pushed-in faces, such as bulldogs, pugs and boxers. In these breeds, or mixes of these breeds, the condition is often associated with—

- Abnormalities of the larynx (area of vocal cords) or pharynx (area behind the nose) that obstruct airflow.
- Abnormally small trachea (windpipe).
- Loud or noisy breathing even at rest.
- Overly narrow nasal passages.
- Soft palate (back half of the roof of the mouth) that extends too far in the throat.

Laryngeal Paralysis. The larynx or vocal cords are paralyzed, so they can't effectively move out of the way when the dog breathes in. This is most common in larger breed dogs. The dog will make loud breathing noises when breathing in or inhaling as opposed to exhaling. Signs may be worse when excited or during warmer months.

Collapsing Trachea. The rings of the trachea collapse into the airway when the animal breathes. It is most commonly seen in small or toy breed dogs of any age. Other causes of upper airway disease or obstruction include airway foreign body, airway tumor and bacterial or viral infection (i.e., tracheobronchitis or kennel cough).

What You Can Do.
1. Check the dog's ABCs; perform CPR as needed. (See CPR, page 36.)
2. Allow the animal to assume the most comfortable position in which to breathe.

3. Transport to the nearest veterinary hospital. Carry your pet, if possible, or use a carrier or box.

Broken Back or Neck

A broken back or neck in a dog is a very serious injury. Your dog may be in extreme pain so it's very important to carefully muzzle him to protect anyone who's trying to help. (See How to Approach, Capture, and Restrain a Dog, page 28.)

Signs and Symptoms.
- Front legs may be stiff and extended
- Dog is in pain
- Anus is open
- Dog may be unable to move his head, hind legs or both front and hind legs
- Dog may dribble urine or feces
- You may see a divot (an area on the spine that appears lower than the rest of the back)

What You Can Do.
1. Check the dog's ABCs; perform CPR as needed. (See CPR, page 36.)
2. Try to slide a board under your dog, keeping him as still as possible.
   - Place a board up on its side along the back of your dog. **(Step 2A)**
   - It is best if the head, chest and legs can be held to prevent movement.
   - Then lower the board and, at the same time, slide the dog onto it, keeping the body and

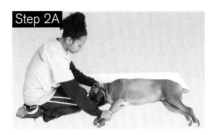

head as still as possible. **(Step 2B)**
- Secure your dog to the board by placing tape or torn strips of cloth over him and around the board. **(Step 2C)**
- Transport him to a veterinary hospital immediately. **(Step 2D)**

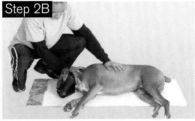

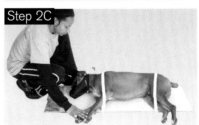

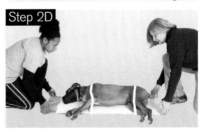

First Aid Reference Guide

Bruises

Bruises may not be obvious, but if your dog is favoring one side or another, she could have one.

Signs and Symptoms. Hematoma (blood-filled swelling) or seroma (serum-filled swelling) under the skin, red to purple marks on the skin, swelling

The Most Common Causes. Bleeding disorder, cancer, mild blunt trauma (i.e., bumping into something)

What You Can Do.
1. Discuss the appearance of the bruised area with your veterinarian.
2. Apply cool compresses to the area four or five times a day for 15 minutes until the swelling goes down (may take several days for a seroma or hematoma).
3. Bruising can also indicate a clotting problem. If you have any question about the cause of the bruising or if there are multiple bruises, take your dog to a veterinarian.

Burns (Major and Minor)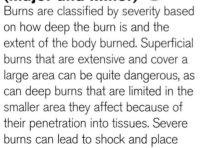

Burns are classified by severity based on how deep the burn is and the extent of the body burned. Superficial burns that are extensive and cover a large area can be quite dangerous, as can deep burns that are limited in the smaller area they affect because of their penetration into tissues. Severe burns can lead to shock and place

your dog at risk for significant infection and potential death.

Burns Involving Only the Superficial Layers of Skin
Superficial burns generally heal well with veterinary care.

Signs and Symptoms. Loss of fur, reddening of the skin, swelling, tenderness or pain

Burns Involving Deeper Layers of the Skin
Deep burns usually heal well, but there may be some skin scarring.

Sign and Symptoms. Blisters, loss of fur, redness, swelling, tenderness

Burns Involving All Layers of the Skin, as Well as Blood Vessels
Deep burns involving blood vessels often heal with a lot of scarring. Intensive care and even surgery may be required.

Signs and Symptoms. Loss of skin, skin is not sensitive to touch, swelling under the skin

Burns in Which the Tissues and Cells of the Skin Are Destroyed
Severe burns result in severe scarring. Intensive medical and surgical care is required.

Signs and Symptoms. Area looks charred (black and leathery)

What You Can Do.
1. Check for the signs of shock in the case of deep or extensive burns. (See Shock, page 102.)

2. Cool water should be applied as soon as possible. This decreases pain and may decrease the penetration of heat further into the tissues. If the burn involves only one body part, you can immerse your dog in a cool bath.

3. If more than one body part is affected, do not immerse your pet. Instead, run cool water directly over the areas or place cool compresses on the areas. Immersing a dog with extensive burns may cool the skin too quickly and cause shock.

4. Place a sterile nonstick pad or clean moist cloth over the burned area to keep it clean.

5. Take your dog to a veterinary hospital immediately.

NOTE: Do not place any ointments, butter or petroleum jelly on burns.

Car Accidents

Dogs are unpredictable at times. Even the best-trained dog can be lured into the street by a cat or squirrel. So always keep your dog under your control either through reliable fencing or a leash. And when travelling in the car, use a dog carrier or special harness available at your pet supply store.

If your dog is hurt in a car accident, check below to see what you can do to help, and take your dog to a veterinarian immediately to check for internal injuries.

The Most Common Causes.
• Getting loose from your yard or a leash
• Being allowed to roam free and running into the path of a vehicle
• Jumping out the window of a car
• Jumping, falling or being thrown from the bed of a pickup truck
• Being run over while you are backing out of the driveway

What You Can Do.
1. If you have witnessed the event, make a mental note of exactly where on the body your dog was hit, whether your dog was simply hit or was driven over and whether your dog was thrown. Often, even in very serious cases, a dog will get up and attempt to walk away. This does not necessarily mean he is not severely injured; it is an instinctive response that makes the dog try to escape danger.

2. Approach the scene cautiously. Alert oncoming traffic. If traffic has not stopped, try to take your dog safely to the side of the road before examining her. It's preferable to always place a muzzle on your dog. If you do not have time to assess how best to carry the dog based on the injuries, simply drag the dog by the fur on top of her body, trying to keep the body as still as possible. Otherwise, follow the steps in the section Carrying and Transporting Techniques, page 32. Take care to not worsen any obvious fracture or limb displacement.

3. If your dog cannot move or appears to have a spinal injury, place her on a flat board for transport. (See Broken Back or Neck, page 59.) If you cannot find a board, use a blanket or shirt (slide your dog onto it and have one or two people hold it on each side as stiffly as possible). If the dog cannot move, she may have a broken back or severe internal injuries, and she may be in shock.
4. Assess and note the following: the position of the dog and the presence of blood, urine or feces (the veterinarian will need this information when you get to the hospital).
5. Does your dog have an open airway, and is she breathing? Or is her breathing labored? Is there a heartbeat or pulse? If not, see CPR, page 36.
6. If alert and standing, observe whether your dog is limping or favoring one side. Look for blood, open wounds, bruising or limbs hanging in abnormal positions.
7. If your dog is bleeding, see Bleeding, page 48.
8. Check for shock. (See Shock, page 102.)

Any dog that has been hit by a car should be taken directly to a veterinary hospital. Many internal injuries caused by the trauma may not show up for 12–72 hours after the incident. These can include slow leakage of blood from internal organs,

rupture of the urinary bladder or other internal organs and air or blood leaking into the chest cavity. Because the dog's body is initially attempting to compensate for the trauma, early shock may be difficult to identify.

Prevention.
- ALWAYS be sure to look around and under your car before backing up.
- NEVER transport your dog in the back of an open pickup truck unless your dog is confined in a sturdy, well-ventilated carrier that is secured to the truck.
- KEEP your dog as an indoor pet and make sure she is leashed while outdoors.

Choking
See Choking in Respond to a Breathing or Heart Emergency, page 38.

Close Encounters (Skunk, Porcupine)
Dogs who are allowed to roam freely might encounter certain wildlife—such as skunks or porcupines—that can lead to very unpleasant experiences. To avoid this problem, be sure to keep your dog on a leash.

Skunk
If your dog encounters a skunk, you will never forget the smell. Although being sprayed isn't life threatening to your dog, the skunk

spray can irritate his eyes and even yours. The smell is difficult to remove and gets tougher the longer it stays on your pet without treatment. So act quickly!

What You Can Do. You will need to wash the dog in tomato juice or an over-the-counter dog shampoo/degreaser (you can even combine them). It may take several washings.

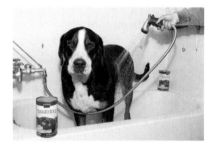

Porcupine
Porcupines, most commonly found throughout the Pacific Northwest and most of North America, are vegetarian rodents known for their unique coat, consisting of about 30,000 quills. Contrary to popular belief, porcupines do not shoot or eject their quills. When they feel threatened, tiny muscles in the skin make the quills "stand up" in defense. A swipe of their tails leaves a bunch of needle-like quills in whatever the tail happens to touch.

What You Can Do. If your dog has only a few quills, and you are certain none are embedded in the mouth or throat, you can try to

remove them with a pair of pliers. However this will be a painful experience for your dog, so have someone help you restrain him.

1. Cover your dog's eyes so he doesn't see the pliers approaching and speak to him in soft, soothing tones.
2. Firmly grab the quill with the pliers close to the skin. Your dog might jerk backward, separating himself from the quill.
3. If there are numerous or deeply embedded quills, or if quills affect your dog's eyes, mouth or throat, take him to your veterinarian immediately where he will have the benefit of anesthesia and pain medications during the removal procedure.

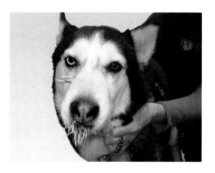

Collapse
A dog that collapses is in serious trouble. She may be in shock, have adrenal gland disease or be beginning to have a seizure. Regardless of the cause, assess your dog to see if she needs CPR, and take her to a veterinarian immediately.

Signs and Symptoms.
Extreme (profound) weakness, sudden falling over, loss of consciousness

The Most Common Causes.
- Abnormal heart rhythm
- Anemia
- Occasionally a primary orthopedic or neurological problem leading to not wanting or being able to get up
- Diabetes (See Diabetes Mellitus in Blood Sugar Emergencies, page 53.)
- Difficulty breathing
- Disease of the adrenal glands
- Heart disease (See Heart Disease and Cardiac Emergencies, page 81.)
- Kidney or liver failure
- Severe blood loss—external or internal into the abdominal cavity (i.e., from a ruptured tumor of the abdomen), into the gastrointestinal tract, into the sac around the heart, into the chest cavity or into the area around the kidneys
- Seizures (See Seizures, page 101.)
- Shock (See Shock, page 102.)

What You Can Do.
1. Check the dog's ABCs; perform CPR as needed. (See CPR, page 36.)
2. Check for shock. Care for shock if needed. (See Shock, page 102.)
3. Take your dog to a veterinary hospital immediately.

Constipation
Even your furry family member can become irregular from time to time. Most of the time, it's nothing to worry about. But in some instances, a dog may have colitis, which is an acute or chronic inflammation of the membrane lining the colon. It causes straining while defecating and mimics constipation. So if the constipation goes on for more than 24 hours, take your dog to the veterinarian.

Signs and Symptoms.
- Crying while straining to defecate
- No stool for more than 1 day
- Small amounts of very hard stool

The Most Common Causes.
- Change in daily routine
- Colitis
- Dehydration
- Eating something inappropriate
- Excessive grooming or eating hair
- Firm/hard stool
- Not eating
- Tumors

What You Can Do. If your dog is still passing stool but it appears to be very firm and he is otherwise healthy (normal eating and drinking), try to add ¼ teaspoon of fiber (such as canned pumpkin or bran) to his diet. If adding fiber to the diet does not work, he is straining to defecate or he appears ill, take him to a veterinarian. **Never use commercial enemas made for humans! These may be toxic and deadly to dogs!**

Cuts and Tears (Major and Minor Lacerations)

Lacerations are wounds that cut through the skin to the deeper underlying layers. They may be deep enough to involve underlying veins, arteries, nerves, ligaments, muscles, tendons or even bone. It is crucial to assess your dog's condition and to see the extent of the laceration so you can treat it the right way. If it's minor, you can treat it at home; if it's major and bleeding heavily, take your dog to a veterinarian.

Signs and Symptoms.
- Bleeding (There may be a great deal of bleeding if an artery was cut.)
- Licking or limping
- Open wound (Underlying structures such as ligaments or muscle may be visible.)

The Most Common Causes.
Accidental injury, trauma, animal abuse, animal fights

What You Can Do. First aid depends on the extent of damage, the degree of bleeding and the cause of the laceration. If there is profuse bleeding, do not attempt to scrub the wound, as you will encourage more bleeding. You should flush the wound with large amounts of water or sterile saline solution, pouring it over the wound but not touching the wound. If the bleeding is not excessive, clean the wound. (See Abrasions, page 42.) If the cause is a bite wound, see Bite Wounds, page 47.

1. Check the dog's ABCs; perform CPR as needed. (See CPR, page 36.)
2. Check for shock. (See Shock, page 102.)
3. Stop the bleeding. (See Bleeding, page 48.)
4. Even if there is no bleeding, cover the area with a clean cloth until you get to a veterinarian.
5. Transport to a veterinary hospital, as many lacerations will require sutures/stitches.

Dehydration
Dehydration is the excessive loss of body fluids and can result from fever, vomiting and diarrhea; not eating or drinking; as well as too much heat exposure.

Signs and Symptoms.
- Change in urination habits (more or less)
- Excessive thirst and mouth dryness (i.e., dry, tacky gums)
- Loss of skin elasticity
- Sunken eyes

How to Determine Dehydration
Pull up on the skin at the back of your dog's neck; it should spring back to the normal position immediately (within 1 or 2 seconds). If it doesn't, she is dehydrated. Very old (geriatric) and very skinny dogs are difficult to assess because skin loses some of its natural elasticity

First Aid Reference Guide

with age and malnourishment. It is also more difficult to assess dehydration in obese animals. In these circumstances, feel the gums; if they feel dry and sticky, your dog is probably dehydrated.

NOTE: If she is drooling, gums may feel moist even though she's actually dehydrated.

The Most Common Causes. Excessive heat exposure and illness—not eating or drinking, vomiting, diarrhea, fever

What You Can Do. A dehydrated dog must be taken to a veterinary hospital for treatment to determine why and how severely she is dehydrated. If she is vomiting or not eating/drinking, she will most likely need fluids either under the skin (subcutaneously) or intravenously. If you aren't sure whether your pet is dehydrated, the safest option is to take your pet to the veterinarian for an examination. You might also try to give your dog an electrolyte-replacement drink like Pedialyte®, but only if she's not vomiting.

Dental Disease, Tooth Damage and Mouth Sores

Dogs rarely complain when they have tooth damage or dental disease, but we dog owners sure know how to complain when their breath smells anything but rosy. Although not life threatening, paying attention to the signs of dental

disease and treating your dog's mouth problems now could prevent him from having bigger issues down the line, because infections starting in the mouth could travel through the bloodstream and cause damage to organs.

Signs and Symptoms.
- Bad breath
- Cracked or broken tooth
- Drooling or difficulty chewing
- Plaque buildup that looks brown or yellow in color
- Recessed, reddened gums or sores in the mouth
- Wanting to eat but then refusing to

The Most Common Causes. Accidents, injury, lack of regular dental care

What You Can Do. Brush your dog's teeth regularly. Your vet can show you how and give you toothpaste to use. Many dogs get very used to this and even enjoy it. Have your dog's teeth checked during his regular checkups to determine if they need to be cleaned with an ultrasonic cleaner (similar to the one your dentist uses).

Diarrhea

Considering what dogs can ingest on a daily basis, it's a small miracle that diarrhea—an increase in the amount, fluidity or frequency of bowel movements—isn't more common than it tends to be. However, if it lasts for more than 24 hours, call your veterinarian.

The Most Common Causes. There are many causes of sudden diarrhea, ranging from your dog having eaten something disagreeable to the first signs of severe illness. A sudden change in diet can lead to stomach upset for your pet. A short list of possible causes includes—

- Chronic inflammatory disease (when the walls of the intestines become irritated and nutrients cannot be absorbed)
- Dietary problems (most common), including eating something improper, such as food off the street or human food; a change in regular diet; or intolerance to previously fed food
- Disease of an organ or organ failure, such as liver or kidney disease or *pancreatitis* (inflammation of the pancreas)
- Glandular disease
- Infectious disease (bacterial, viral and fungal infections)
- Parasitic infection (most common in puppies)
- Tumors in the stomach or intestines; cancer in any organ
- Stress
- Toxin or drug ingestion (See Poisoning, page 96.)

What You Can Do.
1. If the diarrhea continues for more than 24 hours; if your dog is very young (under 1 year), elderly (over 10 years) or otherwise sick; or if vomiting is associated with diarrhea, she should be checked by a veterinarian as soon as possible.
2. If the diarrhea contains blood—either fresh (red stool) or digested (black stool)—have your dog examined by a veterinarian.
3. Check vital signs such as temperature (see How to Take Your Dog's Temperature, page 27), mucous membrane color or capillary refill time (see Observe Your Dog's Mucous Membrane Color and Capillary Refill Time, pages 27–28), and check for dehydration (see Dehydration, page 65). If any of these are abnormal, have your dog examined by a veterinarian.
4. Take away any possible culprit, such as a new food or a new toy, whose use coincides with the onset of diarrhea.
5. Switch to a high-fiber, low-fat or bland diet. If diarrhea subsides after 2–3 days on the bland diet, slowly mix in your pet's regular food and wean back to a normal diet over the course of a week. If attempts to wean to a normal diet don't work and diarrhea resumes, have your dog examined by a veterinarian.
6. As long as there is no vomiting, provide as much water as your dog desires, although she should not gulp down too much at one time. In addition, a pediatric oral electrolyte solution (available in the children's section of your grocery store or pharmacy) is a good source of some of the nutrients lost in diarrhea. If your dog will drink

this solution, this may help to decrease the chance of becoming dehydrated. **Do not withhold water from a dog that has only diarrhea (no vomiting) as this will quickly cause dehydration. For animals who are vomiting, see Vomiting, page 111.**

7. Medications should be used only at the onset of diarrhea. **Check with your veterinarian before giving any medications.** If there is no improvement after one use, your pet appears ill or is vomiting or there is any blood in the stool, do not use the medication again.

   - Kaolin/pectin (e.g., Kaopectate®). Dosage: provide at ½ to 1 milliliter per pound of body weight. (Use dose syringe or dropper.) This can be repeated two to three times per day. Be sure there is no salicylic acid/salicylate in the preparation.
   - Bismuth subsalicylate (e.g., Pepto Bismol®). Dosage: provide at ½ to 1 milliliter per pound of body weight, two or three times per day.

Do not give stronger anti-diarrhea agents to your dog without having her examined by a veterinarian. And when taking an animal to the veterinarian because of diarrhea, take a fresh stool specimen, if possible.

Bland Diet
- Mix boiled chicken with skin, fat and bones removed, or boiled chopped or ground meat with the fat drained off, with cooked white rice using a 1-part-meat to 3-parts-rice ratio.
- Special bland or high-fiber (canned or dry) food purchased from your veterinarian.

NOTE: A bland diet should be used as a temporary measure only to control diarrhea or rest the digestive system after vomiting. It does not contain sufficient nutrients as a permanent diet.

Drowning

Even though dogs are generally good swimmers, they can experience near-drowning, especially if they have been heavily exercised before swimming or if they fall through thin ice. Always keep an eye on your dog when near any body of water.

The Most Common Causes.
- Animal abuse
- Boating accident
- Disasters, such as floods
- Falling through thin ice or falling into water from which they cannot escape
- Not being able to exit a swimming pool (if your dog has access to a swimming pool, be sure he knows how and where to get out)

- Small dog left unattended during a bath in the bathtub
- Swimming too far out and getting fatigued or a muscle cramp

What You Can Do.

1. For an unconscious small dog, lift your dog up by the hind legs (you can suspend him if he is small enough) to allow water to come out the nose or mouth.
2. For an unconscious larger dog, lift the hind legs with the front end on the ground so gravity can help expel the water.
3. Lay your dog down, on either side, with the head slightly lowered.
4. Check the dog's ABCs; perform CPR as needed. (See CPR, page 36.)
5. Place a blanket (thermal, if possible) around your dog.
6. Transport to a veterinary hospital immediately.

Even if you revive your dog, an examination by a veterinarian is still necessary because fluid buildup in the lungs, as well as the effects of hypothermia, may result. (See Hypothermia, page 84.)

Ear Problems (Infections, Injuries)

Ear problems are quite common in dogs, especially in dogs with longer, floppy ears like basset hounds and cocker spaniels. Most of the time, the problems are quite harmless and you can treat them at home. But if it's a severe infec-

tion, it could affect your dog's hearing, so it's best to get her seen by a veterinarian.

Bleeding, Ear Flap
What You Can Do.

- Apply direct pressure to the bleeding site with a cloth or piece of gauze for 5 minutes.
- If bleeding absolutely will not stop with pressure alone, a head bandage may be used (see below).

Making a Head Bandage.

1. Place a gauze sponge or other piece of clean cloth over the wound. **(Step 1)**
2. Hold the ear away from the head and wrap with gauze, starting from the tip of the ear and wrapping in a downward fashion.
3. Once you reach the base of the ear, continue around the side of the head. **(Step 3)**
4. Come around the jaw to the other side of the face and head. **(Step 4)**
5. Repeat two or three times and tape down the end of your material. **(Step 5)**
6. Make sure you can place two fingers inside the bandage so it is not too tight or your dog may have difficulty breathing.
7. Watch your dog to make sure there are no breathing difficulties.
8. Take your dog to a veterinarian to see if sutures are needed.

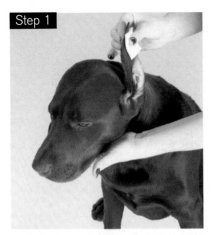

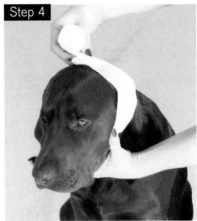

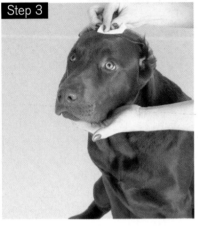

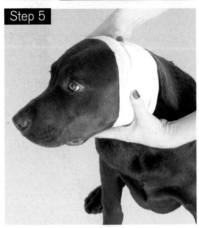

Ear Infections

Ear infections can range in severity from superficial infections to deep infections that can cause hearing loss and balance problems.

Signs and Symptoms.

- Foul odor coming from the ear
- Head shaking or head tilt
- Itching or scratching at ear
- Material in the ear (may be black, brown, white or look like pus)
- Pain when touching the ear
- Red swollen ear, with possible blood

The Most Common Causes.

- Allergies—flea, food or inhalant (pollen, grass, etc.)
- Breed predisposition, especially breeds with long floppy ears
- Ear mites—a common parasite especially in over-crowded conditions (very contagious)

- Infections from bacteria, yeast or parasites
- Water in the ear (from swimming or bathing)

What You Can Do. Have your dog examined by a veterinarian to determine the cause of the ear infection and prescribe the appropriate medication.

Prevention.
- If yeast infections have been diagnosed by a veterinarian, you can help prevent these in the future by cleaning the ear with a mixture of 1 part white vinegar to 10 parts water. Dip a gauze pad into this mixture, and clean ears with it weekly. Only clean the part of the ear that you can see. This helps keep the ear pH low, which discourages and prevents yeast from growing.
- Dry your pet's ear with a gauze sponge after swimming, bathing or cleaning.
- Keep any dog diagnosed with ear mites away from other animals.
- Keep your dog's ears clean.
  - Use gauze sponges to clean ears.
  - Never place cotton swabs into the ear canal. You may push debris further into the ear.
  - Never attempt to go deeper into an ear than you can see.
  - Ask your veterinarian to show you how to clean the ears safely.

Swollen Ear Flap (Aural Hematoma)
An aural hematoma is a collection of blood between the layers of the dog's ear.

The Most Common Causes.
Chronic head shaking from an ear infection, trauma, bleeding disorder

Signs and Symptoms. Swollen, soft and squeezable ear flap and infection (See Ear Infections, page 70.)

What You Can Do. Take your dog to a veterinarian. This condition generally requires the ear flap to be drained surgically.

Prevention.
- Have ear infections treated as soon as they occur.
- If your dog is prone to ear infections, then once or twice weekly clean your dog's ears with a veterinary product that breaks up ear wax. (Ask your veterinarian to recommend the best product for your pet.)

Electric Shock (Electric Cord Bites)
Although not very common, electric shock or electrocution injuries occur when inquisitive dogs bite electric cords. This is more common with puppies.

Signs and Symptoms. Some signs occur immediately; others may not be obvious for hours or even days.

- Collapse on the floor near an electrical cord
- Difficulty breathing and coughing due to a buildup of fluid in the lungs
- Drooling
- Foul odor from the mouth
- Ulcers inside the mouth affecting the tongue, roof, cheek and gums
- Possibly part of the tongue missing
- Loss of appetite
- Shock (See Shock, page 102.)

What You Can Do.
1. Turn off the power, and unplug the cord. If you cannot turn off the power at the source, turn off the power to the house.
2. Check the dog's ABCs; perform CPR as needed. (See CPR, page 36.)
3. Check for shock. (See Shock, page 102.)
4. Take your dog to a veterinary hospital immediately.

IMPORTANT: Do not attempt to free your dog from the cord if the power is on and the cord is still plugged in.

Prevention. None of these techniques are foolproof, but they may help:

- Use plastic sleeves or cord covers to prevent access to electric cords. These are available at hardware or computer stores.
- Place cords in inaccessible locations whenever possible.

- Unplug all electrical cords when not in use.
- Provide appropriate toys for chewing puppies.
- If you see your pet showing interest in a cord, rub the cord with a hot pepper sauce or other deterrents such as Bitter Apple® (available at pet supply stores).

Eye Emergencies
If your dog's eyes are red, she should be examined by a veterinarian to make sure no sight-threatening conditions exist.

Acute Blindness
Acute blindness is most often detected when the dog starts bumping into things, is reluctant to go up or down stairs or is walking gingerly in the surrounding environment.

Signs and Symptoms.
- Bumping into furniture and walls
- Decreased appetite
- Dilated pupils (will look all black) that do not constrict with light
- Other neurological signs like seizures and abnormal behavior
- Reluctance to go up or down stairs or not wanting to walk around

The Most Common Causes.
- Primary eye problems:
  - Chronic disease that appears more acute (i.e., progressive retinal atrophy)
  - Detached retinas, glaucoma, severe corneal ulcers or tumors

- Infection or inflammation inside of the eye
- Primary neurological problems:
  - Primary brain disease (infection, inflammation, tumor)
- Other problems:
  - Low blood sugar

What You Can Do. Any dog with decreased or absent vision should be taken to a veterinarian as soon as possible. In many cases, the primary cause needs to be found and treated to try to preserve vision. Always pay attention to how your pet is acting and if there is a difference in behavior when exposed to dim light vs. bright light.

Cherry Eye—Prolapse of the Third Eyelid Gland

The third eyelid normally sits underneath the lower lid on the side of the eye near the nose. Cherry eye is a swelling and protrusion of the tissue underneath the third eyelid. This condition is more common in young dogs. It is not a true sight emergency but must be distinguished from other eye emergencies.

Signs and Symptoms. The third eyelid comes up and is visible all the time, or it is red and swollen.

The Most Common Causes. Breed predisposition, such as cocker spaniels, and eye infection

What You Can Do. Often this condition will have to be surgically repaired by a veterinarian.

Conjunctivitis

Conjunctivitis is a swelling of the pink tissue lining the inside of the eyelids (conjunctiva). The conjunctiva can be seen by pulling down the lower eyelid and pulling up the upper eyelid.

Signs and Symptoms. The eye has a watery, mucus or pus discharge, and it appears painful, itchy, red and/or swollen.

The Most Common Causes.
- Allergies, chemical irritation or a foreign object in the eye
- Defects in the eyelids (predisposed in some breeds)
- Infection (bacterial, viral or fungal)—especially common in young animals and can be contagious to other dogs or cats
- Lack of tear production

What You Can Do. Have your dog examined by a veterinarian as soon as possible.

Eye Out of Socket (*Proptosis*)

Signs and Symptoms. One or both eyes bulging out of their sockets or other signs of trauma or pain

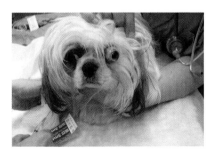

The Most Common Causes.
These injuries are most often caused by trauma (i.e., hit by car, bite wounds). They can, however, be caused by overly aggressive holding of the neck or pulling of collars, particularly in dogs with small snouts and big eyes, like the Pekingese.

What You Can Do.
1. Administer sterile eye wash or sterile petroleum-based eye ointment (artificial tear preparation; available in pharmacies) to help keep the eye from drying out while transporting your dog to a veterinary hospital.
2. **Transport your dog as soon as possible to a veterinary hospital.** There may be significant head trauma that occurred with the proptosis. A veterinarian will decide whether it is feasible to try to put the eye back versus removing it. If the eye is put back, it is to try to save the eye—not the vision.
3. Do not place a leash around your dog's neck. Carry your pet, if you are able. Or you can place the leash under one front leg.
4. Keep your dog from pawing or scratching at the eye.

Foreign Objects in the Eye
Foreign objects are most commonly found on the cornea (the outer layer of the eye) or the conjunctiva.

Signs and Symptoms.
• Obvious foreign object
• Pawing at an eye

• Red or runny eyes, squinting or swelling

The Most Common Causes.
The most common foreign objects in the eye are pieces of plant material, but there are many other objects that can get lodged in the eye. Normally, objects enter the eye either from flying debris or from brushing against a plant.

Flying debris can injure dogs that hang their heads out of car windows. Keep your dog safely inside any moving vehicle. Never transport pets in the back of open pickup trucks unless your dog is confined in a sturdy, well-ventilated carrier that is secured to the truck.

What You Can Do.
1. Gently wash the eye with large amounts of either tap water or sterile saline eye wash. (See Administering Eye Medications, page 12.) Sterile saline eye wash is preferable; it is available at any pharmacy and should be a part of your first aid kit. (See Pet First Aid Kit, page 18.)
2. Inspect the eye with a good light source to ensure the entire foreign object is gone.
3. Even if you are able to remove the foreign object, you should contact your veterinarian. Many foreign objects can cause a corneal ulcer or lead to infections.

Your veterinarian may prescribe topical antibiotics.

If you are unable to remove the object with a stream of liquid, if it appears to be perforating the eyeball or if the eye looks very irritated, take your pet to a veterinary hospital immediately.

Glaucoma

Glaucoma is increased pressure inside the eye caused by a build-up of fluid.

Signs and Symptoms.

- An apparent change in vision
- Cornea may be cloudy
- Eye appears enlarged or pupil may be dilated
- Dog lacks appetite, is lethargic, whines or cries (acute glaucoma may be very painful)
- Pupils unequal in size
- Red or runny eyes
- Dog sensitive to light or squints

The Most Common Causes.

- Breed predisposition (cocker spaniels, basset hounds, samoyeds)
- Displaced eye lens
- Infection or inflammation inside of the eye

The diagnosis of glaucoma must be made by a veterinarian. It involves measuring the pressure inside the eye with an instrument called a tonometer.

What You Can Do. Acute glaucoma is a medical emergency; take your dog to a veterinary hospital immediately. Your pet will probably have to stay in the hospital to receive topical and intravenous medications to reduce the pressure in the eye in order to save the dog's vision. Many animals may eventually require surgery to correct glaucoma.

Ulcers, Corneal

Corneal ulcers are defects on the outer layer of the eye. Dogs with pushed in noses and bulging eyes are very susceptible to getting a corneal ulcer. Breeds like pugs, Boston terriers, Lhasa apsos, Pekingese and Shiz Tzus are some of the most susceptible.

Signs and Symptoms.

- Cloudiness over the eye
- Discharge (watery, mucus or pus)
- May see the defect in the cornea
- Pain, redness, sensitivity to light or squinting

The Most Common Causes.

- Decreased tear production
- Eyelashes that grow inward
- Foreign object
- Infection (bacterial, viral or fungal)
- Masses (tumors) on the eyelids
- Scratch, usually from another animal

What You Can Do. Corneal ulcers are extremely serious. If left untreated, they can affect vision, rupture and cause the loss of the eye. Here is what to do:

First Aid Reference Guide

1. Take your dog to a veterinary hospital immediately.
2. Prevent your dog from rubbing the eye. You may want to use a special device called an Elizabethan collar. (See Elizabethan Collars, page 14.) These are available from your veterinarian or pet supply store. It fastens around your dog's neck and extends around your dog's head like a cone. The purpose is to keep him from rubbing or scratching the eye.

Fading Puppy Syndrome

Fading puppy syndrome usually occurs in the first few weeks of life. The exact cause is not known, and there probably are many factors involved. Unfortunately, it is associated with a high mortality rate.

Signs and Symptoms.
- Cannot keep temperature elevated even with heat source
- Diarrhea
- Low blood sugar leading to wobbliness and decreased mentation
- Not active, gaining weight or nursing/eating

The Most Common Causes.
- Congenital abnormalities
- Inadequate nursing
- Infection—viral and/or bacterial
- Sick mother

What You Can Do.
1. Ensure that the mother is healthy, up to date on vaccinations and receives adequate nutrition.
2. Ensure that the puppy is getting enough nutrition/nursing adequately. Add puppy milk replacer through a bottle if necessary.
3. Weigh puppy daily to ensure she is gaining weight.
4. Make sure room temperature is correct (puppies cannot maintain body temperature for the first few weeks).

Falling (High-Rise Syndrome)

High-rise syndrome most commonly occurs in urban settings due to the risk of falls from tall buildings. Small dogs that can fit through railings are especially at risk for this condition.

Signs and Symptoms.
- Broken teeth
- Difficulty breathing—commonly due to air leaking from a damaged lung
- Fractures or dislocations of the limbs
- Jaw fractures
- Shock and internal injuries
- Split in the roof of the mouth

The Most Common Causes.
Animal abuse; falling or jumping from a window, terrace or other significant height

What You Can Do.
1. Survey the area for safety as you approach.
2. If your dog is not visible, check the entire area around the fall site, including bushes, brush and under cars.

3. Approach the dog cautiously.
4. Check the dog's ABCs; perform CPR as needed. (See CPR, page 36.) Take particular care when opening the mouth, because a jaw fracture may be present.
5. Control any bleeding. (See Bleeding, page 48.)
6. Check for shock. (See Shock, page 102.)
7. If emergency intervention is not needed on the spot, transport to a veterinary hospital immediately.
8. Your transport technique must take into account the suspected injury. A box or carrier to keep the dog in a small, enclosed area is best. (See Carrying and Transporting Techniques, page 32.)

Prevention.
• Always keep screens securely fastened on open windows.
• Don't allow dogs on terraces or balconies that are not screened, except under close supervision.
• Don't leave windows open wide enough for your pet to squeeze through.

Fever
See How to Take Your Dog's Temperature, page 27.

Fishhook Injuries/Penetration
Dogs are curious creatures. They often explore with their noses; if they smell an already-used fishhook, they may ingest the hook thinking there are fish remnants on it or they may eat a fish with a hook in its mouth. The most likely places for fishhooks to be found are around the face and muzzle, inside the mouth and on the paw. It is also possible for a dog to swallow a fishhook whole.

Signs and Symptoms.
• Fishhook protruding from the skin; fishing line protruding from the mouth or anus
• Loss of appetite, painful mouth or excessive drooling

The Most Common Causes.
• Accidental injury
• Playing with or sniffing fishing equipment
• Swallowing a baited hook

What You Can Do. Your dog should be taken to a veterinarian for hook removal. If it is not possible to get him to a veterinarian immediately, try the following:

1. Push the hook through the exit wound until the barb is visible.
2. Cut the barb off with a wire cutter.
3. With the barb removed, pull the hook out backwards, the way it went in.
4. Treat like a wound. (See Puncture Wounds and Embedded Object, page 99.)
5. Even if you successfully remove the hook, take your dog to a veterinarian for wound assessment and possible antibiotic therapy.

First Aid Reference Guide

If the hook is embedded inside the mouth, or if fish line is attached to a hook and swallowed, immediately transport your dog to a veterinary hospital where surgery may be performed. **Do not attempt to pull out the hook!**

Foreign Objects (Skin, Eye, Mouth, Nose, Throat, Swallowed)
Skin

Splinters and thorns are common foreign objects, as are sticks and glass. They can be found anywhere on dogs, but are frequently embedded in the pads of their feet.

Signs and Symptoms.
- Bleeding
- Licking at a paw
- Not placing any weight, or placing less weight, on a limb
- Obviously protruding thorn or other object
- Swelling at the site of the foreign object

The Most Common Causes.
- Accidental injury
- Encounter with a porcupine (See Close Encounters, page 62.)
- Running into a sharp object such as a stick or fence

What You Can Do.
1. Sterilize a pair of tweezers and a needle, either by passing them through a flame or by dipping them in an alcohol solution.
2. Direct a good source of light to the area.
3. With the ends of the tweezers, take hold of and pull out the object. If it breaks, or if there are deep fragments, particularly of glass, do not attempt to remove them. Take your dog to a veterinary hospital for removal.
4. If the splinter is just below the surface of the skin, try to scrape the overlying skin with the needle, and then grasp the object with the tweezers.
5. After removing the object, soak the affected area in a dilute solution of warm (not hot) water and Epsom salts for 15 minutes. Repeat this three or four times daily until the healing is complete.
6. If the wound is deep, if you cannot remove the entire object or if your dog does not put weight on the limb, take your dog to a veterinary hospital.
7. Also see Puncture Wounds and Embedded Object, page 99.
8. Discuss the injury with your veterinarian. Antibiotics may be required.

Run your hands lightly over your dog's head, body, legs and feet every day to check for foreign bodies, injuries or parasites. Your dog will love the extra contact and affection!

Eye
See Eye Emergencies, page 72.

Mouth

Sticks are notorious for getting lodged in the roof of a dog's mouth. If you see your dog pawing at his mouth, that could be the problem.

The Most Common Causes. The most common causes of injury are from sticks or toys.

Signs and Symptoms. Drooling, not wanting to eat, pawing at the mouth

What You Can Do. Look inside your dog's mouth and check the roof of the mouth. Try to get the object out with your fingers, but if she seems distressed, call your veterinarian. It may require sedation to remove the object.

Nose

Objects can become lodged in the nose, most commonly in hunting dogs.

The Most Common Causes.
Blades of grass, grass awns, sticks

Signs and Symptoms. Nasal discharge, sneezing excessively

What You Can Do. Supervise your dog while outside.

Throat
See Choking, page 62.

Foreign Objects Swallowed
Signs and Symptoms. Refusal to eat, vomiting

The Most Common Causes.
• Eating corn cobs, marrow bones, other human food
• Ingesting articles of clothing
• Swallowing toys

What You Can Do. It may be a wait-and-watch situation as some foreign bodies will pass through the digestive tract, but don't take any chances. Call your veterinarian first to see if inducing vomiting (by the doctor) is feasible. Otherwise, it may require endoscopy or surgery.

Frostbite
Sure, your dog has fur to help protect her from the elements, but that doesn't mean she can't succumb to frostbite, which is actually the freezing of a body part or exposed skin and is a common occurrence in cases of acute hypothermia (See Hypothermia, page 84.). The body parts most susceptible to frostbite include your dog's tail, tips of the ears and the pads of the feet. In the winter, be sure to clean your dog's feet after a walk to remove road chemicals, salt and ice particles to help protect her from frostbite.

Signs and Symptoms.
• Discoloration of the frozen area; skin that is pale or even blue in color initially, looking black and dead in later stages
• Lack of pain or sensation at the affected area or a lot of pain, especially when the area starts to warm up

The Most Common Causes. The causes of frostbite are the same as those for hypothermia. (See Hypothermia, page 84.)

What You Can Do.
1. Take your dog out of the cold.
2. Spray the affected area with warm water.
3. Lightly apply a warm compress to the area (ensure it is not hot enough to cause a burn). Do not rub or apply pressure to the area as that could worsen the damage.
4. Transport your dog to the nearest veterinary hospital for care and to assess the affected area to see if there is permanent damage. If the tissue is dead, local amputation may be necessary.

Gunshot Wounds

Thankfully, gunshot wounds are not a common occurrence for man's best friend. However, they can happen accidentally if your dog enjoys hunting with you. If he does get shot, assess him, perform CPR, if needed, and get him to a veterinarian immediately.

Signs and Symptoms.
- Lameness/fractures
- Profuse bleeding
- Signs of an entrance and/or exit wound
- Stumbling and falling to the ground

What You Can Do.
1. Your dog may attempt to run away; keep him as calm as possible.

2. Any part of the body may be affected, so it is important to examine him carefully and thoroughly. You may see a wound where the bullet penetrated, or it may be difficult to find because it is covered by fur. Additionally, there may be a second wound where the bullet exited the body.
3. Check the dog's ABCs; perform CPR as needed. (See CPR, page 36.)
4. Try to stop the bleeding and cover obvious wound sites with gauze, a nonstick dressing or a clean cloth, and hold it in place. (See Bleeding, page 48.)
5. Check for shock. (See Shock, page 102.)
6. If the bullet has penetrated the chest and your dog is not breathing, perform rescue breathing (see CPR, page 36) and cover the chest wound with gauze or other clean material. These materials can be wrapped around the chest. Ensure that the wrap is not too tight to constrict chest movement.
7. With as little movement as possible, transport your dog to a veterinary hospital immediately.

Head Entrapment

Dogs can accidentally get their heads stuck in plastic or glass jars, leading to suffocation.

What You Can Do.
1. If it's a plastic jar, support the jar and head and use scissors or a screwdriver to punch holes

in the jar so that the animal can get oxygen. You can also try to cut the jar in half.

2. If it's a glass jar, support the jar and head and gently tap the glass or use a hammer to break the glass so your dog can breathe.

3. Once there are holes or openings in the jar, use wire cutters, cardboard scissors or other scissors to cut off the rim of the jar. If possible, place a towel between the dog's neck and the rim.

4. Once the jar is off, if the dog is not breathing, check her ABCs and perform CPR as needed. (See CPR, page 36.)

5. Transport the dog to a veterinary hospital for evaluation. Suffocation, even for a small amount of time, can lead to fluid buildup in the lungs, requiring oxygen therapy.

Prevention. Keep all jars, particularly those that contain food, away from dogs.

Heart Disease and Cardiac Emergencies

Heart disease is quite common in dogs, with one of the most telltale signs being a cough. Although heart disease and cardiac emergencies are serious, if you catch them early enough, your dog will benefit. (See also Respond to a Breathing or Heart Emergency, page 35.)

Signs and Symptoms.
• Bloated belly
• Coughing, especially when lying down
• Decreased tolerance for exercise
• Fainting, particularly following exercise or from heat exposure (Often the dog will look disoriented or drunk and fall over. This behavior is different from a seizure. The easiest way to tell is to check your dog's gum color. If it is white or very pale, it is probably a fainting episode. If the gum color is pink or red, it is probably a seizure. Also, during a seizure the dog will tend to be less responsive and not know who you are.)
• Increased breathing rate or breathing difficulty
• Jugular veins (in the neck) may become enlarged
• Loss of appetite

The Most Common Causes.
• Abnormal heart rhythm
• Breed predisposition (Certain breeds of dogs and mixes of these breeds are particularly susceptible to heart problems. For example, toy poodles and other small dogs may have problems with their heart valves and certain large-breed dogs, such as Doberman pinschers and boxers, are more prone to dilation and weakening of the heart muscle.)
• Cancer
• Cardiac birth defects
• Endocrine disorders such as hypothyroidism in dogs

First Aid Reference Guide

- Enlargement or dilation of the walls of the heart
- Improper nutrition
- Infections such as canine parvovirus and heartworm disease

What You Can Do.
1. Check the dog's ABCs; perform CPR as needed. (See CPR, page 36.)
2. Check for shock. (See Shock, page 102.)
3. Take your dog to a veterinary hospital immediately.

Prevention.
- Feed your pet a high-quality food.
- Take your pet for his yearly regular veterinary checkups; it's the best way to find and follow up on heart murmurs or abnormalities.
- Keep your dog up to date on heartworm testing and preventive medication. Heartworms can live in the heart of dogs. The infection transmits from one animal to another by mosquitoes. Left untreated, heartworm infection almost always leads to heart failure, but it is easy to test for and prevent. Ask your veterinarian for more information!

Heat Stroke (Hyperthermia) and Heat Exhaustion

Heat stroke, or hyperthermia, occurs when a dog severely overheats—most commonly in the spring and summer months—when the weather turns warm and the dog has not yet acclimated to it. The good news is if the heat stroke hasn't advanced too far (with a body temperature of more than 104° F), you can help your dog recover.

NOTE: Dogs don't have sweat glands, so they can dispel heat only by panting and through the pads of their feet. Make sure your pet has plenty of cool water and shade during hot weather.

Signs and Symptoms.
- Collapse
- Body temperature 104° F or above (See How to Take Your Dog's Temperature, page 27.)
- Bloody diarrhea or vomit
- Capillary refill time that is too quick (See Capillary Refill Time, page 28.)
- Depression, stupor (acting drunk), seizures or coma
- Excessive panting or difficulty breathing
- Increased heart rate (See Heart Rate and Pulse, page 24.)
- Increased respiratory rate (See Breathing Rate, page 26.)
- Mucous membrane color is redder than normal (See Observe Your Dog's Mucous Membrane Color, page 27.)
- Salivation

The Most Common Causes.
- A previous episode of heat stroke
- Breed predispositions (Dogs with short snouts, such as bull-

dogs, are particularly susceptible to hyperthermia.)

- Dog left in a parked car
- Dog not acclimated to the warmer weather
- Excessive exercise in hot, humid weather (This may be exercise that your dog can usually handle, but not in the warmer weather.)
- Lack of appropriate shelter for an animal outdoors
- Prolonged seizures
- Thick-coated dogs in warm climates
- Underlying disease state, such as upper airway, heart or lung disease

IMPORTANT: Never leave your pet in a parked car! Even with the windows cracked, your pet can quickly suffer heat stroke–and even die. Temperatures can exceed 120° F in parked cars!

What You Can Do.
1. Get your dog out of direct heat.
2. Check for shock. (See Shock, page 102.)
3. Take your dog's temperature. (See How to Take Your Dog's Temperature, page 27.)
4. Spray your dog with cool water. If using an outdoor hose, run the water for a minute or so to cool it off before spraying your pet. Spray him for a minute or two, then retake his temperature.
5. Place water-soaked towels on the dog's head, neck, feet, chest and abdomen.

6. Turn on a fan and point it in your dog's direction.
7. Rub isopropyl (rubbing) alcohol 70% on the dog's foot pads to help cool him. Do not use large quantities of alcohol (more than half a pint), as it can be toxic if ingested by dogs.
8. Immediately take your dog to the nearest veterinary hospital.

NOTE: The goal is to decrease the body temperature to about 103° F in the first 10–15 minutes. Once 103° F is reached, you must stop the cooling process because the body temperature will continue to decrease and can plummet dangerously low if you continue to cool the dog.

Even if you successfully cool your pet down to 103° F, you must take him to a veterinarian as soon as possible because many consequences of hyperthermia won't show up for hours or even days. Some of these conditions can be fatal if not treated medically. Potential problems include—

- Abnormal heart rhythms.
- Destruction of the digestive tract lining, leading to bloody vomiting and/or bloody diarrhea.
- Kidney failure.
- Neurological problems, including seizures and swelling of the brain.
- Problems with blood clotting.
- Respiratory arrest.

First Aid Reference Guide

Hot Spots

Hot spots are inflamed areas of the skin caused by your dog licking, biting or scratching the skin too much. Most of the time, they are found on the legs or hind end but can occur at any site on the body. They can have different degrees of severity depending on how long your dog has been aggravating the area. Typically, the lesions start as red or pink bald patches from your dog's biting and may end up bleeding and infected. So the earlier you catch them, the better for your dog.

Your dog may be creating a hot spot because she is bored. Combat boredom by providing her with safe toys she really enjoys, as well as exercise and lots of hugs and attention.

Signs and Symptoms. Bleeding in the area, red or pink bald patches, discharge or foul odor from the area

The Most Common Causes.
- An area that may have originally been irritated by a sting, an external parasite such as a flea, a foreign object, a scrape or an allergic condition
- Food allergies
- Psychological causes, such as boredom

What You Can Do.
1. Shave the area with grooming clippers.
2. Clean the area with warm water.
3. Look for the presence of any foreign objects, including insect stingers or fleas, and remove them.
4. Apply a topical, over-the-counter, triple antibiotic and steroid cream or ointment, although more severe hot spots may not respond as well.
5. Try putting an Elizabethan collar on the dog. (See Elizabethan Collars, page 14.) You can buy one from your veterinarian or a pet supply store. These collars fasten around your pet's neck and extend around the head like a cone. This keeps the dog from biting at most parts of the body and will prevent her from licking the topical treatment. Dogs don't like wearing them, but they can help dramatically.
6. If topical treatments don't work, have your dog examined by a veterinarian.

Hypothermia (Dangerous Drop in Body Temperature)

Hypothermia is a drastic reduction of body temperature and happens when dogs have been exposed to frigid temperatures for too long or if the fur gets wet in a cold, windy environment. When the body temperature drops, the heart rate and breathing slow down. The consequences of extreme hypothermia include neurological problems (including coma), heart problems, kidney failure, slow or no breathing and frostbite. (See Frostbite, page 79.)

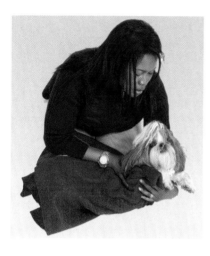

Signs and Symptoms.

- Body temperature below 95° F (See How to Take Your Dog's Temperature, page 27.)
- Decreased heart rate (See Heart Rate and Pulse, page 24.)
- Pale or blue mucous membranes (See Observe Your Dog's Mucous Membrane Color, page 27.)
- Pupils that may be dilated (The black inner circle of the eye appears larger.)
- Shivering
- Stupor, unconsciousness or coma
- Weak pulse

The Most Common Causes.

- Falling into cold water or not being acclimated to the cold weather
- Shock
- Stray or outdoor animal caught in the cold or a storm without shelter

- Underlying illness
- Inability to regulate body temperature (seen in very old and very young dogs)

What You Can Do.

1. Remove your dog from the cold.
2. Check the dog's ABCs; perform CPR as needed. (See CPR, page 36.)
3. Assess for shock. (See Shock, page 102.)
4. Take a rectal temperature. (See How to Take Your Dog's Temperature, page 27.)
5. Wrap your dog in a blanket. (See Pet First Aid Kit, page 18.)
6. Place warm water bottles next to the dog, wrapping the bottles in towels to prevent burns.
7. Transport to a veterinary hospital immediately.

Insect Bites

See Allergies and Allergic Reactions, page 42; Parasitic Disease, page 91; and Venomous Bites and Stings (Snakes, Scorpions, Toads and Jellyfish), page 109.

Kennel Cough

Kennel cough causes a very dramatic, dry cough and is very contagious. Often, it will resolve on its own; however, treatment may be necessary in severe cases.

Signs and Symptoms.

- Dry, hacking cough; may be slightly productive

- May progress to pneumonia; symptoms include:
  - Anorexia
  - Lethargy
  - Difficulty breathing
  - Nasal discharge
  - Fever (See Know What's Normal, page 24.)

The Most Common Causes.
- *Bordetella bronchiseptica* is the underlying bacterium that causes classic kennel cough. It hinders the normal tracheal mechanisms that protect the airway and lungs, which can lead to severe pneumonia that may be difficult to treat.
- The dog may have other secondary bacterial infections or a viral infection.

What You Can Do.
1. Put the dog in a bathroom filled with steam for 10–15 minutes three to four times a day.
2. Talk to your veterinarian about over-the-counter vs. prescription cough suppressants.
3. If your dog develops signs consistent with pneumonia or the cough is not resolving after about 5 days, take her to a veterinarian.
4. If the dog develops pneumonia, then she will require antibiotics. Puppies are especially at risk of developing pneumonia and will most likely require intravenous antibiotics, along with fluids and oxygen therapy.

Prevention.
- Keep your new puppy away from other puppies and dogs, especially at kennels and dog parks.
- Talk to your veterinarian about vaccinating against *Bordetella.* Do not vaccinate right before the animal is being kenneled or some other stressful event. Vaccinate at least 1 month prior to needing it (most kennels require vaccination).

Mammary Glands (Swollen or Red)
Mammary glands are on the underbelly of a dog from the front armpits to the back legs and in females are used to feed puppies. When mammary glands are swollen, painful or red, the condition is called mastitis and is usually due to a blocked milk duct. It may occur in female dogs when they feed their puppies. Female dogs can also develop mammary gland tumors that can become infected. This condition is not due to nursing and should be examined by a veterinarian.

Signs and Symptoms.
- Decreased appetite, fever, lethargy and vomiting
- Discharge from the gland (may look like milk with blood or pus in it)
- Swollen or red mammary gland that feels hot to the touch

The Most Common Causes.
- Dirty living conditions, infection or trauma from nursing puppies
- Pregnancy
- Tumor

What You Can Do.
1. Clean the nursing environment, including the whelping box, surrounding areas and anything coming in contact with your dog.
2. Place warm compresses on the affected gland every 3 or 4 hours for 10–15 minutes.
3. Have your dog examined by a veterinarian who most likely will prescribe antibiotics if there is an infection.

Prevention. Keep nursing areas and living areas clean and dry. Spay your dogs to prevent pregnancy.

Masses/Skin Swelling/Abscess, Lipoma or Tumor

Dogs can get masses or swellings either in the skin or just under the skin (subcutaneous). Warts and benign masses are common in dogs as they get older.

Signs and Symptoms.
- If in the skin, it can look like a wart or pimple and be soft to firm.
- If under the skin, it can look like a swelling or ball-shaped mass.
- It may have a discharge.

The Most Common Causes.
- Abscess
- Fatty tumor under skin (Called a *lipoma*, it is benign and will feel soft.)
- Malignant mass in skin (mast cell tumor) or under skin

What You Can Do.
1. When petting your dog, feel through the fur coat to find small masses.
2. If one is found, write down where it is, its size and if it is firm or soft.
3. Contact your veterinarian about aspirating the mass (sticking a needle into it to identify the cells and type of mass).
4. Monitor the size and tell your veterinarian if it is changing.
5. An abscess will be soft and the skin will most likely be red, hot and painful. If it has already ruptured, then you might see pus or bloody discharge.
6. For a ruptured abscess, see Puncture Wounds and Embedded Object, page 99, for wound care, and contact your veterinarian. The dog will most likely need antibiotics.
7. If not ruptured, contact your veterinarian.

Nails (Broken or Torn Toenails)

If your dog spends a lot of time outside or walks on pavement regularly, he may need his nails trimmed only occasionally because the contact on rough surfaces helps grind the nails down on their own. But if he enjoys the comforts of home most of the day, he will need regular nail trimming to prevent breaking or tearing. If your dog tears a nail, it will bleed and be painful, but it will grow back. The dew claws (the thumb toes higher on the foot) are very susceptible to tearing because they don't reach the ground and are not subject to normal wear. So be sure to check the dew claws when trimming nails. Regularly clip only the sharp tips of your pet's nails using a clipper designed for dogs. Your veterinarian can show you how.

Signs and Symptoms.
- Bleeding from the toe
- Dog placing less weight on the leg with the broken toenail
- Dog shaking his paw
- Licking

The Most Common Causes.
- Cutting a toenail too short during trimming
- Injury
- Not trimming toenails on a regular basis

What You Can Do. If the nail is bleeding, apply styptic powder to the area. This should be a part of your pet first aid kit. (See Pet First Aid Kit, page 18.) You can also try applying direct pressure to the nail with a piece of gauze or clean cloth for 5 minutes. If you do not have these items available, try the following:

1. Take a bar of soap and push it into the bleeding nail, or apply flour or cornstarch to the area with firm pressure for 5 minutes.
2. If you are not successful, wrap the paw (See Pad Wounds, page 89.) After bandaging the paw, transport your dog to a veterinary hospital.

If you are able to stop the bleeding at home, wait 1 day (to make sure you do not disturb the clot that has formed) then soak the paw in warm water and a saline solution to help it heal. Monitor the site for infection, as

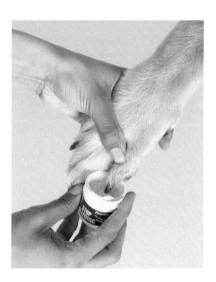

evidenced by swelling, pain, redness and reluctance to put weight on the paw. If any of these signs appear, take your dog to a veterinarian.

Nosebleeds

Usually nosebleeds happen only as a result of injury or blunt trauma, and first aid at home can help get your dog back to good health. However, if there's a small amount of blood leaking from her nostril without evidence of injury, this could be something more serious and she should get to a veterinarian as soon as possible.

Signs and Symptoms. Bleeding from either or both nostrils

The Most Common Causes.
- Bleeding disorder
- Foreign object
- Infection, head trauma or injury
- Tumor

What You Can Do.
1. Apply an ice pack, wrapped in cloth, to the nose.
2. Place steady pressure on the bleeding nostril using a clean cloth or gauze.
3. Keep the dog as quiet and still as possible.
4. If the bleeding does not stop, is the result of anything but simple trauma (such as a thorn in the nose) or there is no obvious reason for the bleeding, take the animal to a veterinarian immediately for an examination. A small

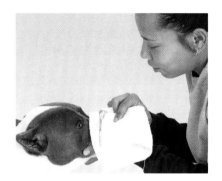

amount of blood from one nostril may be an early sign of a tumor or bleeding disorder.

Pad Wounds

The pads of your dog's feet contain many blood vessels that cause them to bleed heavily when injured. Due to their location and function, injuries are quite common.

Signs and Symptoms.
- Bleeding (may be heavy)
- Limping or not putting weight on the limb
- Wound or foreign object in pad

The Most Common Cause.
Stepping on a sharp object, such as a thorn or a piece of glass

What You Can Do.
1. Remove any obvious foreign object. (See Foreign Objects [Skin, Eye, Mouth, Nose, Throat, Swallowed], page 78.)
2. Wash the area with saline solution (add 1 teaspoon of salt to 1 quart of warm water to make solution) or with warm water alone.

First Aid Reference Guide

3. Dry the foot.

4. Bandage the foot by placing a strip of adhesive tape (see Pet First Aid Kit, page 18) on each side of the foot, starting several inches above the wound and extending several inches past the bottom of the foot. **(Step 4)** The tape on either side of the leg acts like stirrups to hold the bandage in place—the tape should go directly on the fur.

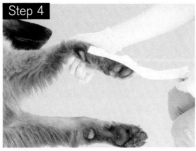

Step 4

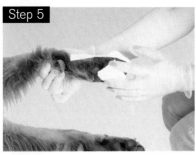

Step 5

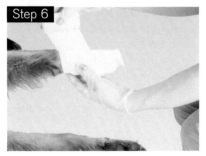

Step 6

5. Place a nonstick pad or gauze sponge over the wound. **(Step 5)**

6. Wrap the paw with gauze roll (in the first aid kit), starting from the toes and ending just above the ankle or wrist. **(Step 6)**

7. Pull the ends of the sticky tape over the end of the gauze roll bandage as far as it will go, with the sticky part twisted to face and adhere to the bandage.

8. Place an elastic or cling roll bandage over the cotton, working from the toes to the ankle. Do not wrap tightly. **(Step 8)**

9. Make sure the bandage is not too tight; check for toe swelling and feel the limb just

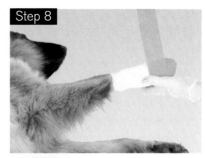

Step 8

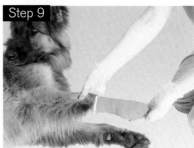

Step 9

above the bandage for coolness, swelling or pain. If any of these are evident, loosen the bandage. **(Step 9)**

10. Transport your dog to a veterinary hospital to get the wound assessed.

Parasitic Disease

Parasitic disease, including chiggers, fleas, intestinal worms, mites and ticks, is not uncommon in dogs. While some parasites don't cause too much concern, some of them can cause chronic disease. Read on about how you can detect and treat these pesky parasites in your pooch.

Chiggers

These are common skin parasites found throughout the central and southern United States. They can bite and infect humans and dogs and cause severe itching. They can be treated relatively easily.

Signs and Symptoms. Itching caused by small, reddish-orange mites about the size of a pinhead, resembling paprika, found on the legs, head and abdomen

The Most Common Causes.
Walking through a chigger-infested area (Chiggers are found in grassy areas, mostly in the spring and fall.)

What You Can Do. Wash your dog with a mild shampoo. Contact your veterinarian about antihistamines or other treatments if severe.

Fleas

Fleas are small, wingless insects with elongated back legs that allow them to jump onto a passing animal host. They feed on the blood of numerous animal species—including humans.

Signs and Symptoms.
- Intense scratching, sometimes accompanied by hair loss, redness and/or raised bumps on the skin
- Adult fleas or "flea dirt" (feces a female flea deposits when laying eggs) visible on dog

NOTE: Use a flea comb and water spray to search for evidence of fleas on your pet's head and hindquarters. Flea dirt will turn red when moistened because it is primarily digested blood.

The Most Common Causes.
- Contact with a flea-infested animal
- Contact with flea eggs, larvae or pupae in your dog's indoor or outdoor environment

What You Can Do. A flea infestation must address each one of the flea's four stages of development: eggs, larvae, pupae and adults. To be effective, you must treat both your dog and his environment.

- Talk to your veterinarian about the best way to treat your dog and other animals in the house.

First Aid Reference Guide

- Thoroughly vacuum your home including behind and under furniture, drapes and your pet's bedding and crate. Afterward, seal the vacuum bag in a plastic bag and discard it right away.
- Treat your home with a product that contains both an adulticide and an insect growth regulator that will kill adult fleas as well as stop the development of eggs and larvae.
- Clean and treat your automobile, garage, basement or any other place your dog frequents.
- Treat yard and kennel areas with an environmentally safe spray. Concentrate on areas where your dog spends most of his time outdoors, such as the patio, under the deck or porch and in and around the dog house. (Depending on the product used, you may need to repeat the yard treatment weekly or monthly.)
- Rake away and dispose of organic debris, such as leaves, weeds and grass clippings, to reduce the flea habitat.
- Be persistent. It may take several weeks or even months to get rid of all of the fleas, in all life stages.
- Contract with a professional exterminator to treat severe infestations.
- Be aware that your dog can have an allergic reaction to a flea infestation. (See Skin

Allergies in Allergies and Allergic Reactions, page 43.)

IMPORTANT: Read the label on all insecticides thoroughly and apply them as directed. Be especially careful if your household includes children, someone with asthma, or pet fish or birds.

Prevention. The easiest and best way to control a flea infestation is to prevent one in the first place. There are a variety of flea control products you can use, including collars, sprays, dips, topical applications, shampoos and powders. There also are oral and injectable medications available. Ask your veterinarian which flea prevention and control method he or she recommends for your pet. Always talk to your veterinarian before using more that one product at a time.

IMPORTANT: Never use an insecticide intended for dogs on a cat.

Intestinal Worms (Roundworms, Hookworms, Whipworms)
Several different types of intestinal worms exist. These worms may be visible in the stool or they may be vomited up (more common in puppies). Roundworms look like pieces of spaghetti and hookworms can lead to significant blood loss if left untreated.

The Most Common Causes.

- Dogs can pass the worms and eggs in their stool or vomit, and can acquire them easily by smelling or eating other animals' feces. It is best to assume that all the pets in a household are infected if one case of roundworms has been positively confirmed.
- Puppies get roundworms directly from their mother's milk when they start to suckle.

Signs and Symptoms.

- Anemia (pale gum color)
- Bloated abdomen
- Diarrhea, vomiting and weight loss
- Loss of appetite, or an animal that is very hungry but not gaining weight
- Poor-looking coat of hair

What You Can Do.

1. Take the animal to a veterinarian along with a stool sample. If you see worms in the vomit or stool, make sure the sample includes the worms.
2. Have your pet's stool checked for worms at his yearly physical examination or sooner if you suspect an infestation.

NOTE: It is very important to treat roundworm infections, as they may be transmitted to humans. Any pet that has been treated for worms should have a follow-up fecal examination to ensure the treatment was successful.

Prevention.

- Don't allow your dog to eat or sniff the feces of other animals.
- Don't introduce a new animal into your household without first having the animal checked and treated for worms.
- Have your pet's stool checked yearly by a veterinarian.
- Remove your dog's stool after defecation.

Mites and Mange

There are 3 different kinds of mange: Demodectic, Cheyletiella and Sarcoptic. Each one is caused by different species of mites—tiny, 8-legged critters related to spiders.

Signs and Symptoms.

- Crusty ear tips
- Hair loss, sometimes spreading throughout the body
- Oozing sores or lesions
- Pin-point bite marks
- Secondary skin infection (in severe cases)
- Severe itching, especially on the elbows, ears, armpits, hocks, chest and abdomen (Mites prefer to live on skin areas with less hair.)
- Small, red pustules
- Yellow crust on the skin

The Most Common Causes.

Sarcoptic mange, commonly known as canine scabies, is caused by the parasite *Sarcoptes scabiei.* These microscopic mites burrow into the skin of dogs or puppies where they lay eggs. Newly hatched mites continue tunneling under the skin. These mites can survive for several days off the host, so dogs can become infected without ever coming into direct contact with an infected dog.

Demodectic mange, also known as red mange, follicular mange or puppy mange, plagues mostly young dogs. It is caused by the mite *Demodex canis,* which is transferred from the mother to offspring in the first few days of life. The first sign, hair loss, usually does not occur until after the puppies are 4 months old. Usually, hair loss begins around the muzzle, eyes and other areas on the head. Sometimes this looks like a few circular crusty areas, usually around the muzzle. In more severe cases, a dog could have generalized infestation all over the body.

Cheyletiella mange, also known as walking dandruff, affects puppies and is caused by a large, reddish mite that can be seen with a magnifying glass. This mange is identified by the dandruff dusting that occurs over the dog's head, neck and back. It causes mild itching. Walking dandruff is highly contagious but short-lived. The mite that causes the mange dies soon after leaving the host.

What You Can Do. Mange can easily be mistaken for other skin conditions, making it impossible for pet owners to diagnose accurately.

If your dog suffers from irritated, itchy skin, make an appointment with the veterinarian. Early diagnosis will give you a head start on a cure. Your veterinarian can prescribe topical, oral or injectable medications for mites.

In addition to treating the infestation itself, the veterinarian may prescribe antihistamines and steroids to help relieve your dog's itching. Antibiotic treatment also may be needed if a secondary infection has developed.

Ear Mites. The mite *Otodectes cynotis* takes up residence in an animal's ear canal. It is highly contagious and causes intense itching of the ears.

Signs and Symptoms.
- Scratching around the ears and/or frequent head shaking
- Fresh or dried blood visible inside the ear canal

NOTE: Dried blood resembles coffee grounds in the ear canal. If you notice this, your dog probably has ear mites.

Most Common Causes.
- Contact with another animal that has ear mites

What You Can Do.
- Check your dog's ears regularly for any discharge or redness.
- Talk to your veterinarian about how to safely clean your dog's ears at home.

NOTE: Your dog can have an allergic reaction to mites. (See Allergies and Allergic Reactions, page 42, and Ear Problems, page 69.)

Tapeworms

Tapeworms are commonly spread when an animal bites an itch or eats fleas that harbor tapeworm larvae.

Signs and Symptoms.

- Round or flat small white worms that look like moving pieces of rice, which are segments of the tapeworm body, will be seen around the anus or in the stool.
- For other signs, see Intestinal Worms, page 92.

What You Can Do. Practice flea control, and have your dog dewormed with medication administered by a veterinarian. Clean your animal's bedding thoroughly after starting treatment for tapeworms.

Ticks and Tick-Borne Diseases

Ticks are blood-sucking parasites responsible for the transmission of several diseases to dogs, cats and humans. They commonly jump on animals as the animals walk through tall grass or brush against leaves, bushes and trees. To get the most accurate information for your area, ask your veterinarian about diseases transmitted by ticks.

Signs and Symptoms of Tick Infestation.

- A tick may appear as a tiny dark-colored insect or a fat, skin-colored bump; it is engorged with the dog's blood and has its head burrowed into the dog's skin.
- Ticks may be present anywhere on the body, but they are commonly found on the ears (or just inside them) and on the feet or legs.
- The area around the tick may be red and swollen.

The Most Common Causes of Tick-Borne Diseases. Tick-borne diseases (i.e., ehrlichia, Rocky Mountain spotted fever, babesiosis, Lyme disease) can cause a variety of illnesses, some of which can be life threatening. These diseases can lead to paralysis, anemia, low platelet count, joint pain and swelling, and fever.

What You Can Do.

- If you live in an area that has ticks, or after visiting such an area, check your pet thoroughly. Run your fingers through your pet's entire hair coat; check the paws by lifting each up and inspecting the pads; look between the toes and inside the floppy part of the ear.
- If you find a tick—
  1. Put on nonlatex gloves.
  2. Place a small amount of tick spray (available in pet stores or at your veterinary

First Aid Reference Guide

hospital) on a gauze sponge, cotton ball or paper towel and hold it over the tick. This will usually cause the tick to start to back out in 30–60 seconds.

3. When the tick starts to back out, grab the entire tick with a pair of tweezers.

4. Alcohol, mineral oil or petroleum jelly can be used in place of the tick spray, but they generally don't work as well. Don't use matches to singe the tick, as it may burn the animal's skin.

5. Flush the tick down the toilet or, if you are not sure what type of tick it is, you may want to save it in a secure container for identification by your veterinarian. (Different kinds of ticks carry a variety of diseases communicable to animals and humans.)

6. Apply a disinfectant such as alcohol or an antibiotic ointment to the site of the tick bite. A local skin reaction may occur around where the tick was attached.

Prevention. There are many products available for the prevention of ticks. Before using a tick product, check with your veterinarian to ensure it is safe for your dog's size and age. Also, ask your veterinarian if a Lyme disease vaccine is right for your dog.

Poisoning

Because many plants can be poisonous to pets, ask your veterinarian which plants may be poisonous to dogs or check the American Society for the Prevention of Cruelty to Animals' (ASPCA's) Web site (*www.aspca.org/toxicplants*) for a list of poisonous plants. Better yet, before adding plants to your home or garden, assume that a plant can be harmful unless you know it is not.

If you suspect your dog has been exposed to any type of poison, call your veterinarian first. Then, if needed, contact the Animal Poison Control Center at 888-426-4435, 800-548-2423 or 1-900-680-0000 for advice on what to do.

Signs and Symptoms. Poisons can be eaten, inhaled or absorbed through the skin. The signs of poisoning may occur immediately or within hours, or may take days to appear. They include—

- Bleeding from anus, mouth or any body cavity.
- Dilated pupils.
- Salivation (drooling or foaming at the mouth).
- Seizures or other abnormal mental state or behavior, such as hyper-excitability, trembling, depression, drowsiness or coma.
- Shock. (See Shock, page 102.)
- Swollen, red irritated skin or eyes.

- Ulcers in the mouth or burned lips, mouth or skin.
- Vomiting or diarrhea (with or without blood or particles of the ingested toxin).

The Most Common Causes.

- Accidental ingestion
- Animal abuse
- Eating food that may be toxic to a dog
- Eating garbage
- Giving improper medication to a dog without understanding the consequences

Sources of Toxins

- Antifreeze (ethylene glycol)
- Drugs such as marijuana, cocaine, amphetamines and alcohol
- Heavy metals (i.e., zinc, lead)
- Household chemicals, including cleaning solutions, chlorine, lead-based paint and potpourri
- Household foods, including chocolate, onions, moldy cheese, raisins and grapes
- Inhaled toxins such as carbon monoxide
- Many plants, both indoor and outdoor
- Non-prescription drugs such as acetaminophen (Tylenol®), aspirin, ibuprofen (Advil®) or cold remedies
- Prescription medications, either prescribed for your dog and taken in inappropriate dosage or belonging to someone else in the household and accidentally eaten by the dog

- Rat or mouse poison/bait or other pesticides, snail or slug bait, moth balls
- Topical products such as flea powders, sprays, shampoos and dips—especially those containing pyrethrins, carbamates and/or organophosphates

What You Can Do.

1. Check the dog's ABCs; perform CPR as needed. (See CPR, page 36.)
2. Check the mucous membrane color. (See Observe Your Dog's Mucous Membrane Color, page 27.) Certain toxins cause specific changes in the color. For instance, cherry-red mucous membrane color occurs in cases of carbon monoxide poisoning.
3. Check the capillary refill time. (See Capillary Refill Time, page 28.)
4. Check the animal's mental state, looking for seizures, increased excitement, unsteadiness, depression or coma.
5. Call your veterinarian or veterinary emergency hospital. Your veterinarian may have you call the ASPCA's Animal Poison Control Center (888-426-4435) before coming to the hospital.

In either case, have the following information on hand, if possible:

- Exact name of the poison
- How much the animal ate or was exposed to

First Aid Reference Guide

- How long ago the exposure or ingestion occurred
- The animal's vital signs (temperature, heart rate, breathing rate, capillary refill time and mucous membrane color)
- Approximate weight of the animal

At home, you will only be able, at best, to assist in ridding the pet's body of the toxin, depending on the type of poison. For specific types of poisoning, follow the information below.

Topical Poisons

1. Call your veterinarian or the ASPCA's Animal Poison Control Center for information about the specific poison involved. Before washing your dog, make sure that it is safe for her to get wet, as water may activate some poisons.
2. Always wear nonlatex gloves. If allowed, wash the animal with large volumes of water. If your pet is having a reaction to a flea product, a mild hand soap or baby shampoo can be used. For oil-based toxins (such as petroleum products), use dishwashing liquid.
3. If the poison is in the eye, flush the eye with large volumes of water or sterile eye wash. (See Administering Eye Medications, page 12.)
4. If the poison is a powder, you will need to dust or vacuum it off.

Inhaled Poisons

Gases, such as carbon monoxide, can cause poisoning.

1. Take your dog into fresh air as quickly as possible.
2. Perform rescue breathing as needed. (See CPR, page 36.)
3. Check for shock. (See Shock, page 102.)

IMPORTANT: To protect your family, including your pet, install a carbon monoxide detector in your home.

Ingested Poisons

It may be appropriate to induce vomiting, but **DO NOT induce vomiting until you speak with a veterinarian or the ASPCA's Animal Poison Control Center.** With some caustic substances, it may be appropriate to give your dog milk to help absorb the poison, but this should be decided on a case-by-case basis. Let your veterinarian or the Animal Poison Control Center advise you.

DO NOT induce vomiting if your dog–

- Is having difficulty breathing.
- Is experiencing seizures, depressed or acting unusually excited.
- Is unconscious.
- Has a history of bloat.
- Has a very slow heart rate. (See Heart Rate and Pulse, page 24.)

Or if–

- The toxin is suspected or known to be a caustic substance (such as a drain opener), an acid (such as from a battery) or a petroleum-based product.
- The object eaten was sharp or pointed.
- The poison container says not to do so.

How to Induce Vomiting

If your veterinarian or the ASPCA's Animal Poison Control Center gives you the okay to induce vomiting, you can give household (3 percent) hydrogen peroxide orally, 1 teaspoon per 10 pounds of body weight. (See Giving Your Dog Medication, page 11.) Repeat this every 15–20 minutes, up to three times, on the way to the veterinary hospital.

Syrup of ipecac can be dangerous to dogs and should NOT be used to induce vomiting, unless specifically advised by your veterinarian.

If you are not sure what your pet ate, take the vomit to the hospital with you. If you know what the substance was, take the vomit and the container the toxin was in. **In any case of poisoning, take your pet to the veterinary hospital as soon as possible.**

- If you are unable to induce vomiting, the animal's stomach may need to be pumped.

- If ingestion occurred some time ago and the toxin has already been partially absorbed, blocking further absorption is the next step. This may include giving the pet activated charcoal.
- A few toxic substances have antidotes. To determine an antidote, the veterinarian must know what the animal ate.
- Depending on the poison, there may be serious bodily consequences, including organ failure, and the dog must be treated by a veterinarian with intravenous fluids and medications.

Puncture Wounds and Embedded Object

Puncture wounds can look minor from the outside, but can be deceptively deep and serious. If the wound is not immediately apparent, the injured dog may develop an infection 1 or 2 days after injury.

Signs and Symptoms.

- Bleeding
- Evidence of an embedded object
- Evidence of infection—redness, swelling, discharge, pain
- Small wound in skin (If there are two puncture marks, this is a good indication the wound was caused by a bite. For how to properly treat a bite wound, see Bite Wounds, page 47 and Venomous Bites and Stings (Snakes, Scorpions, Toads and Jellyfish), page 109.

- Bruising (If this occurs, there may also be significant internal injury to both muscles and organs.)

The Most Common Causes.
Animal abuse, injury from a pointed object

What You Can Do.
1. If the wound is bleeding excessively, control the bleeding. (See Bleeding, page 48.)
2. Check the dog's ABCs; perform CPR as needed. (See CPR, page 36.)
3. Check for shock. (See Shock, page 102.)
4. Administer basic wound care. (See Abrasions, page 42.)
5. If there's an embedded object and it does not appear to penetrate into deep tissues, you can try to remove it with sterilized tweezers, taking care not to push it deeper inside. You should then contact your veterinarian to determine when the wound should be evaluated.
   - If the object appears deeply embedded, do not attempt to remove it. Take the dog to a veterinarian as soon as possible; he may need immediate surgery or intervention once the object is removed.
6. If your dog is ill and has an abscess that has not ruptured, take him to a veterinarian as soon as possible for abscess care.

7. If your dog has an abscess that has ruptured, clean the area as described under Abrasions, page 42, and take him to a veterinarian.

Puppy Strangles
Puppy strangles, also known as juvenile cellulitis, usually occurs between the age of 3 weeks and 4 months. The reason for the name is that the lymph nodes under the jaw or chin become enlarged and look as though they might strangle the puppy. However, once puppy strangles is detected, the prognosis is quite good.

Signs and Symptoms.
- Anorexia (refusal to eat)
- Enlarged lymph nodes (glands) under the chin, which are painful
- Fever
- Joint pain
- Pustules (little abscesses) and granulomas on face and ears
- Swollen face (lips, muzzle and eyelids)

The Most Common Cause.
An immune disorder with a genetic component

What You Can Do.
1. Administer basic wound care. (See Abrasions, page 42.)
2. Take your dog to a veterinarian to determine if there is a bacterial or infectious cause. In either case, she will then need oral steroids with or without antibiotics.

Rectal Prolapse

If your dog strains to defecate, and you see a red, sausage-shaped mass pushing out of his anus, he may have rectal prolapse. This is an emergency, so get him to a veterinarian as soon as possible. The earlier it's caught, the better the outcome for your dog.

Signs and Symptoms. Pain; red, sausage-shaped mass out of the anus; straining

The Most Common Causes.

Diarrhea; chronic straining to defecate and/or urinate; pushing during whelping (giving birth)

What You Can Do.

1. Lubricate the area with a sterile, water-based lubricant.
2. Take your dog to a veterinarian immediately. Depending on the extent of the rectal prolapse, the veterinarian will have to move it back in place and suture the area to make the opening smaller. If the tissue is not viable or healthy, surgery may be needed.

Prevention. If your dog is persistently straining to defecate or has persistent diarrhea, contact your veterinarian to determine the underlying cause and start treatment.

Seizures

As terrifying as they may be to watch, most seizures don't harm your dog. Many have no residual effects at all. But if it's your dog's first seizure, take her to a veterinarian as soon as possible for an evaluation. If it's not your dog's first seizure, but her seizures last longer than 2 minutes or there are multiple, repeating seizures, take her to the veterinarian immediately. This is a medical emergency.

Signs and Symptoms. Phases of a seizure:

- Before a seizure (pre-ictal), your dog may seem dazed or anxious, may seek you or seek a safe place.
- During an active seizure (ictal), the animal often will fall over, twitch, urinate, defecate and drool. In addition, she may not recognize you or may fall over and be stiff and rigid (grand mal seizure). Some seizures may look like the dog is just staring into space or biting at invisible things (chewing gum seizures).
- After a seizure (post-ictal), the animal may be disoriented, walk into walls or appear to be blind. Dogs may also behave normally following a seizure.

The Most Common Causes.

Central nervous system causes include the following:

- Abscess
- Epilepsy
- Infection in the brain (bacterial, fungal, viral or parasitic)
- Inflammation in the brain
- Malformation of the brain (birth defect)

First Aid Reference Guide

- Scar tissue in the brain (may occur after a head injury)
- Tumor

Non-central nervous system causes include the following:

- Glandular disease causing blood sugar to be too low or too high (as may occur in diabetics)
- Low blood calcium
- Organ failure, particularly of the liver and kidney, which are the waste treatment plants of the body (When they malfunction, a large build-up of toxic waste products can occur, causing seizures.)
- Poisoning—such as from certain drugs, plants, lead, heavy metals, antifreeze and chocolate

The seizure's cause must be identified to determine if the collapse was due to primary respiratory, heart, orthopedic or neurological problems.

What You Can Do.
1. Make sure your dog is in a safe place (not on top of a staircase or anywhere from which a fall is possible).
2. Record how long the active phase of the seizure lasts.
3. Keep a log of your dog's seizures. Include the date, time of day, time after a meal and how long the active seizure phase lasts.
4. Keep your hands away from the animal's mouth. Do not attempt to hold your dog's tongue (the

animal will not swallow her tongue). Your dog may not know who you are during a seizure. Many pet owners are bitten while attempting to handle their pets during a seizure.
5. Do not disturb your dog during and after an active seizure.
6. If this is your pet's first seizure, call your veterinarian. Your dog should be examined as soon as possible.
7. Seizures lasting longer than 2 minutes or cluster seizures (seizures repeated one after the other) are medical emergencies; these animals are at risk for very high fevers and brain damage. A veterinarian must examine an animal having cluster seizures immediately.

NOTE: If your dog is placed on anti-seizure medication, understand that the medication does not cure the cause of the seizure; it simply helps to reduce the number or severity of episodes. Your dog will probably have future episodes and require frequent veterinary checkups.

Shock
See also Respond to a Breathing or Heart Emergency, page 35.

Shock is a body's response to a change in blood flow and oxygen to the internal organs and tissues. This can result from a sudden loss of blood, a traumatic injury, heart failure, severe allergic reaction (anaphylactic shock), organ disease or an infection circulating through the body (septic shock). There are three stages of shock, which may look very different.

Early Shock
The body attempts to compensate for the decreased flow of fluids and oxygen to the tissues.

Signs and Symptoms.
- Body temperature that may be low or elevated
- Capillary refill time of 1–2 seconds (See Capillary Refill Time, page 28.)
- Increased heart rate (See Heart Rate and Pulse, page 24.)
- Mucous membranes that are redder than normal (common with septic shock)
- Normal to increased intensity of pulses (may feel like they are pounding)

Middle Stages of Shock
The body begins to have difficulty compensating for the lack of blood flow and oxygen.

Signs and Symptoms.
- Cool limbs
- Depressed mental state
- Hypothermia (low body temperature of less than 98° F) (Hairless areas may feel cool to the touch.) (See Know What's Normal, page 24.)
- Increased heart rate (See Heart Rate and Pulse, page 24.)

- Pale mucous membranes
- Prolonged capillary refill time (See Capillary Refill Time, page 28.)
- Weak pulse

End Stage or Terminal Shock
This occurs when the body can no longer compensate for the lack of oxygen and blood flow to its vital organs.

Signs and Symptoms.
- Depressed mental state or unconsciousness
- Prolonged capillary refill time (See Capillary Refill Time, page 28.)
- Slow respiratory rate (See Heart Rate and Pulse, page 24.)
- Slow heart rate (See Heart Rate and Pulse, page 24.)
- Weak or absent pulse

IMPORTANT: Cardiopulmonary arrest may soon follow! Prepare to perform CPR. A dog that is in shock, or that you suspect may be in shock, should be taken to a veterinary hospital immediately.

What You Can Do.
1. Assess the dog's ABCs; perform CPR as needed. (See CPR, page 36.)
2. Control bleeding if present. (See Bleeding, page 48.)
3. Warm the animal with a thermal blanket. (See Pet First Aid Kit, page 18.) Wrap the blanket around the animal's body.

First Aid Reference Guide

4. Elevate the hind end slightly by placing a blanket underneath the hind end. **NOTE: Do not do this if you suspect a broken back.** (See Broken Back or Neck, page 59.)
5. Take your dog to a veterinary hospital immediately.

Slipped Disc (Intervertebral Disc Disease)

A slipped disc or intervertebral disc disease occurs when a disc (the cushiony material between each of the vertebrae of the spine) becomes damaged and presses on the adjacent spinal cord. This can happen in the dog's neck (cervical spine) or over or behind the ribs (thoracic or lumbar spine). Although it can occur in any dog, it's more common in smaller breeds, especially in dachshunds, cocker spaniels, beagles and miniature or toy poodles. Larger dog breeds can have a slipped disc in the neck or back, but a clot in the spinal cord (called *fibrocartilaginous emboli*) could also cause the symptoms. The cause must be determined by an MRI or myelogram.

Signs and Symptoms.
- Arched back stance
- Crying in pain, even without being touched
- Evidence of trauma
- Trembling
- Very painful back or belly
- Lack of control while urinating or defecating
- Inability to walk, rear legs that may collapse or show some degree of paralysis, stumbling, dragging of feet or toes
- Not putting head down to eat or drink
- Not wanting to go up or down stairs

The Most Common Causes.
- Breed predisposition
- Injury/trauma

What You Can Do.
1. Take your dog to a veterinarian as soon as possible. Carry the animal or restrain in a carrier, cage or on a board. (See Carrying and Transporting Techniques, page 32.)
2. If complete paralysis occurs, your pet may need surgery to walk again.
3. If paralysis is partial, your veterinarian may prescribe anti-inflammatory medications. Once you give these, you must confine your pet in a cage or crate because the anti-inflammatory medication will make your dog feel better and more inclined to move around. This could potentially worsen his condition. An animal should be crate-rested for 4 weeks (usually longer than the medication is given).

Prevention. Especially in breeds that are predisposed to a slipped disc, discourage any jumping on or off furniture, beds, etc.

Smoke Inhalation

Smoke inhalation is a life-threatening emergency and needs veterinary attention immediately. In fact, smoke can be more deadly than burns. Dogs who inhale smoke will gasp or cough and may stop breathing. Moreover, many smoke inhalation consequences may not be apparent for days. So, if your dog is exposed to fire or smoke, take her to the veterinarian immediately for an evaluation.

Signs and Symptoms.
- Abnormally fast breathing (See Breathing Rate, page 26.)
- Cherry-red gums, in the case of carbon monoxide poisoning
- Coughing
- Discharge from the mouth or nose
- Eye discharge
- Labored breathing
- Stopped breathing
- Singed hair with a smoky odor on the coat

What You Can Do.
1. **Immediately remove dog from smoke and into fresh air.**
2. Check the dog's ABCs; perform, as needed. (See CPR, page 36.)
3. Check for shock. (See Shock, page 102.)
4. Take your dog to a veterinary hospital immediately.

Some of the life-threatening consequences include—

- Body fluid and electrolyte imbalances.

- Corneal ulcers or damage to the eye surface.
- Fluid accumulation in the lungs or chest cavity.
- Pneumonia.
- Swelling of the mouth and throat.

Sneezing

It is normal for dogs to sneeze occasionally. While sneezing itself is not serious, if it is persistent, excessive or accompanied by nasal discharge, it might be a symptom of other health problems that should be addressed by your veterinarian. Depending on the cause, sneezing could be accompanied by a clear, pussy or bloody nasal discharge.

The Most Common Causes.
Allergy, bleeding disorder (such as a problem with blood clotting), congenital defect, foreign object in the nose or tumor

Reverse Sneezing
Dogs occasionally have episodes of reverse sneezing, which is not a medical emergency. The dog inhales and suddenly has a reverse snort. Several snorts in a row may look very dramatic, but as soon as the reverse sneezing stops, the dog immediately acts normally. Although the cause is unknown, post-nasal drip is often the culprit. Reverse sneezing typically occurs suddenly, as an isolated incident. There is no need to seek veterinary care unless the animal does not return to normal

First Aid Reference Guide

within a few seconds after stopping or seems to be in respiratory distress. If the episode continues, check for shock. (See Shock, page 102.)

Strangulation

See also Respond to a Breathing or Heart Emergency, page 35.

The most common cause of dog strangulation is being leashed inappropriately or becoming tangled when tied to a stationary object. If your dog is strangled, it's important to make sure he's breathing and, if not, start CPR immediately.

Signs and Symptoms. Choking, gasping for air

The Most Common Causes. Abuse, entanglement, leashes or collars getting caught on objects, pulling too hard on a leash

What You Can Do.
1. Check the airway and start CPR, if indicated. (See CPR, page 36.)
2. An animal that becomes strangled or pulls too hard on a leash is at risk for respiratory distress from a fluid build-up in the lungs (nonheart failure edema), which can take a few hours to develop.
3. Always take any dog showing signs of strangulation or that has been strangled to a veterinarian as soon as possible.

Suffocation

See Head Entrapment, page 80, and Respond to a Breathing or Heart Emergency, page 35.

Tail Swelling/Injury

While this is not a life-threatening emergency, tail injuries and swelling are common in dogs and can be painful.

Signs and Symptoms. Bloody tail, holding tail awkwardly, licking or biting tail

The Most Common Causes.
• Abscess/wound
• Exercise or swimming (These can cause inflammation and pain.)
• Trauma (i.e., tail caught in a door, car accidents, an animal bite)

What You Can Do.
1. Gently examine the area to see if it's red and inflamed. If it is, see Abrasions, page 42, and Bite Wounds, page 47.
2. Take your dog to a veterinarian who may take an x-ray to rule out a fracture. If the area remains inflamed, your doctor may prescribe an anti-inflammatory medication. If there is an abscess, antibiotics will be prescribed. If there is a laceration or cut, sutures may be needed.

Testicular or Scrotal Swelling

In intact male dogs, the testicles or the scrotum (the sac that holds the testicles) can swell from injury or a condition called *testicular torsion*, a life-threatening emergency. It is important to get your dog to a veterinarian as soon as possible to determine the cause.

Signs and Symptoms. Anorexia, extreme pain, lethargy, redness, swelling

The Most Common Causes.
• Bites from other animals
• Burns
• Cuts
• Frostbite
• Testicular torsion (testicle twisting around vessels)
• Tumor

What You Can Do.
1. Check for shock. (See Shock, page 102.)
2. Take your dog to a veterinarian immediately to have testicular torsion ruled out. If it's not torsion, your dog may have an infection that requires antibiotics and possibly castration.

Prevention. Have your dog neutered. This will help prevent some prostatic diseases as well.

Urinary Accidents/Incontinence

Your dog may be housebroken, then one day have an accident that leads to several more. Or your dog begins urinating during sleep or while lying down, especially spayed

females with weak bladders. In either case, finding the cause with your veterinarian is key.

The Most Common Causes.
• Infection
• Excessive water consumption
• Glandular disease
• Neurological disease
• Steroids like prednisone (These will make the dog urinate more and drink to compensate.)
• Weak bladder (sphincter)—more common in spayed females

What You Can Do. Although it's not life threatening, the best thing to do is call your veterinarian as soon as you notice two sequential accidents. The doctor will be able to determine the cause and possibly prescribe medication.

Urinary Blockage

Urinary blockage is a medical emergency and can result from a stone or bladder or urethral disease. If left untreated, the body will begin to reabsorb the waste products normally removed by the urine—this build up quickly becomes toxic. In addition, the bladder can tear easily after being stretched for prolonged periods and may even rupture. If you suspect a urinary blockage, do not attempt to feel the bladder yourself, as it may be very delicate and may rupture from even the gentlest touch!

Signs and Symptoms.
• Blood in the urine
• Coma

- Crying, particularly when a dog tries to urinate
- Crying to be walked frequently
- Depression (hiding, unresponsive or refusing food)
- Excessive licking of the genital region
- Frequent, small volume of urine
- Lethargy
- Loss of appetite
- Slow heart rate
- Squatting to urinate with nothing or only small drops present, and frequent squatting in the same outing
- Swelling of the genital region
- Vomiting

The Most Common Causes.
- Prostate disease
- Tumor
- Urinary stone

What You Can Do.
1. **You must take the animal to a veterinary hospital immediately! This is a medical emergency!**
2. If your dog is small (less than 30 pounds), carry him by holding the body behind the back legs so you don't place pressure on the bladder. You can also place your pet in a box or carrier.

At the hospital, with your dog under sedation, a catheter will be placed into the bladder to wash it out and allow the animal to urinate. Some animals need surgery to remove the obstruction or stones, if present.

Prevention.
- Finish all antibiotics or other medication prescribed for a urinary tract problem, as the condition may persist for long periods even after your dog seems better.
- Strictly adhere to special diets prescribed for a dog with a history of urinary blockage, bladder infection or stones.
- Always make sure your dog actually passes urine and is not just squatting or lifting his leg unproductively.

Vaginal Discharge and Uterine Infection

Unspayed female dogs are at risk for uterine infections. The infections generally occur as she gets older and has gone through many heat cycles. These tend to flare up a few weeks to a month following a heat cycle. Less commonly, infections at the site from which the uterus was removed in spayed females also occur.

Signs and Symptoms.
- Discharge from vulva (This may look bloody or may look like pus and have a foul odor. Some uterine infections will not have a discharge due to the cervix being closed.)
- Increased drinking and urination
- Lethargy
- Licking at vulva area
- Loss of appetite
- Vomiting

The Most Common Cause.
Bacterial infection, which causes a buildup of pus in the uterus

What You Can Do. Take your dog to a veterinary hospital immediately. This condition is an emergency and must be dealt with at once, or the uterus may rupture.

Prevention. Spay female dogs to reduce the risk of infection.

Venomous Bites and Stings—Snakes, Scorpions, Toads and Jellyfish

Snakebites
Poisonous snakes in the United States include—

* **Pit vipers–**These include rattlesnakes, copperheads and cottonmouths. Pit vipers have a depression between their nose and eyes. Their fangs can retract and their heads are triangular in shape.
    * **Rattlesnakes** can be up to 8 feet in length; tails contain a rattle.
    * **Copperheads** are about 4 feet long and have no rattles. The top of the head is a rich, coppery orange color.
    * **Cottonmouths**, also known as water moccasins, can grow to 4 feet in length. The body is dark, and the inside of the mouth is snowy white.

* **Coral snakes–**These snakes have fangs that are in the rear of the mouth and are not retractable. They can be up to 3 feet long. They are red, yellow and black in alternating bands.

Signs and Symptoms.
* Bleeding puncture wound
* Blood does not clot
* Breathing stops
* Bruising or sloughing of the skin over the bitten area
* Fang marks may or may not be visible, due to dog hair
* Neurological signs such as twitching and drooling
* Pain
* Reddening
* Signs of shock
* Swelling of the bitten area; can be severe and progress for more than a day

What You Can Do.
1. If you suspect a poisonous snakebite, attempt to identify the snake, but don't get too close. If you have to kill the snake to protect yourself or your pet, take it with you for identification. **Be aware that the fangs on a decapitated snake's head may be venomous for up to 1½ hours.**
2. Check the dog's ABCs; perform CPR as needed. (See CPR, page 36.)
3. Check for signs of shock. (See Shock, page 102.)
4. Attempt to keep the animal calm and still.

5. Put on nonlatex gloves and wash the wound with water and mild soap. **Do not cut open the wound or attempt to suck out the venom! Do not place ice on the area or use a tourniquet!** (Depending on the situation, such actions may do more harm than good.)

6. Immediately transport your dog to a veterinary hospital. If possible, carry your pet to the car. Any movement may cause the toxin to spread faster.

7. Some non-poisonous snakes may also bite. This bite may cause an allergic reaction. If your pet is bitten by a non-poisonous snake, treat it as you would a puncture wound (see Puncture Wounds and Embedded Objects, page 99, and or Bite Wounds, page 47) and watch for allergic reactions. (See Allergies and Allergic Reactions, page 42.) If you are unsure if the snake was poisonous, follow steps 1–6.

Scorpions

Although most scorpion bites are not deadly, being bitten is an emergency, especially since a sting from the more rare bark scorpion can be fatal. Get your dog to a veterinarian immediately if a scorpion sting is suspected.

Signs and Symptoms.
- Accidental urination and defecation

- Breathing problems
- Collapse and potentially death
- Dilated pupils
- Drooling
- Pain
- Paralysis
- Swelling
- Tearing from the eyes

The Most Common Causes.
Curiosity

What You Can Do. Take your dog to a veterinarian immediately for treatment.

Toads

The vast majority of toads are not poisonous, but the Colorado River toad (found mainly in the Southwest United States) and the giant brown toad or marine toad (found in Florida, South Texas and Hawaii) can kill a dog within 30 minutes. The poisons on a toad's skin can cause severe discomfort and even paralysis or death. So any time you notice the remains of a toad in your dog's mouth or you've seen your dog licking a toad or its remains, call your veterinarian.

Signs and Symptoms.
- Collapse
- Diarrhea
- Excess salivation
- Fever
- Pawing at the mouth
- Seizures
- Vomiting
- Weakness

The Most Common Causes.
- Licking or eating a toad
- Licking the remnants of where a toad was sitting

What You Can Do.
1. Flush out the dog's mouth with water and look for signs of shock. (See Shock, page 102.)
2. Get your dog to a veterinarian immediately.
3. If it's determined he's been poisoned, it's likely your dog will need to stay overnight at the animal hospital for monitoring with an electrocardiograph and intravenous fluids.

Jellyfish Stings
Definitely not deadly, but if your dog gets stung by a jellyfish he will be in pain and uncomfortable. The good news is most jellyfish stings can be treated with your own first aid.

Signs and Symptoms.
- Pain
- Stingers present
- Swelling

The Most Common Causes.
Getting stung while swimming in jellyfish-inhabited waters

What You Can Do.
1. Pour rubbing alcohol on any tentacles left in the skin. It will help stabilize the toxins.
2. Use sticky tape to remove any jellyfish tentacles from the dog's fur.
3. Make a paste of baking soda and water and apply to

where the stings are to soothe the area.
4. Contact your veterinarian to ask whether you can give diphenhydramine (Benadryl®). (See Diphenhydramine Dosing in Allergies and Allergic Reactions, page 43.)

Vomiting
Vomiting can be scary. While not normal, most of the time it is a temporary condition and your dog will be fine. But if vomiting continues after you withhold food for a day (as long as the dog is an otherwise healthy adult), it could signal a more serious problem; also, your dog will be at risk for dehydration and will have to see a veterinarian immediately. If your dog is not producing any vomit but is dry-heaving, it could signal bloat (see Bloat and Torsion, page 50) and she will need to be rushed to the veterinarian. On the other hand, if your dog vomits intermittently within the time span of a month or several months and has diarrhea and has lost weight, get her checked by a veterinarian, as it could signal inflammatory bowel disease.

The Most Common Causes.
- Bacterial, viral or parasitic infection
- Change in diet
- Eating something that upsets the stomach
- Eating something that cannot pass through the gastrointestinal tract and is stuck, such as a foreign object

First Aid Reference Guide

- Eating toxic materials, including chewing on many types of plants
- Glandular disease
- Linear foreign bodies (i.e., string, rope or panty hose that travels through the stomach and intestines, gets caught, bunches the intestines and saws through the wall of the intestine)
- Motion sickness
- Organ inflammation, infection or failure, such as kidney disease or pancreatitis
- The result of many illnesses

What You Can Do. If your dog is vomiting but otherwise acting normally, then a conservative approach is best. Take the following steps:

1. Give no food or water by mouth for 8–12 hours. Withholding food and water is appropriate only for young adult or otherwise normal, healthy animals. Elderly (over 10 years), very young (under 1 year) or otherwise ill animals should not go without food or water; they should be examined by a veterinarian. Use the following size ranges for food and water rationing after vomiting:
   - Small dog: 20 pounds or less
   - Medium dog: 21-49 pounds
   - Large dog: 61-100 pounds
   - Giant dog: 100 pounds or more
2. If no vomiting occurs while not eating or drinking, offer the animal a small quantity of ice chips and repeat every 2–3 hours as long as vomiting does not recur.
3. If no vomiting occurs with ice chips after 6 hours, add a small amount of water (¼ cup for a small dog, ⅓ cup for a medium dog and ½ cup for a large or giant dog) or a pediatric electrolyte oral solution in addition to the water. Repeat every 2–3 hours if no vomiting occurs.
4. If your dog is still not vomiting after 8–12 hours with the water, add a bland or high-fiber diet (see Bland Diet in Diarrhea, page 68): 2 teaspoons at a time for small dogs; 1 tablespoon at a time for medium-sized dogs; and 2 tablespoons at a time for large and giant dogs. Repeat every few hours as long as no vomiting occurs.
5. During the next 48–72 hours, if no vomiting occurs, increase the amount of food and decrease the frequency. During the next 3–5 days, gradually mix the animal's regular diet with the bland diet, slowly returning to a normal dietary regimen.
6. If vomiting occurs despite withholding food and water, or if vomiting occurs on the reintroduction of food and water, you must take the animal to a veterinarian to rule out more serious and possibly life-threatening conditions and to treat dehydration and nausea.

7. If other signs of illness accompany the vomiting, such as fever or lethargy, do not withhold food and water. Take the animal directly to a veterinarian for examination.

IMPORTANT: Rapid dehydration is possible if the animal is not eating or drinking and is losing body fluids as a result of vomiting and/or diarrhea. Dehydration can lead to shock and death. Giving ice cubes or ice chips instead of water can prevent dehydration and keep a dog from drinking too much water too soon.

First Aid Reference Guide

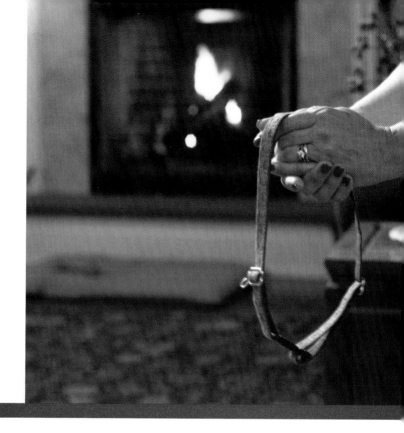

7

When It's Time to Say Goodbye

Chances are you regard your dog as a furry family member. So saying goodbye is certainly not easy. But sometimes, no matter how hard you try, it's just not possible to keep your dog happy and well any longer. Perhaps he is old and in failing health, or he may be young but afflicted with a painful, chronic condition that will worsen over time or perhaps he was involved in a traumatic accident.

Euthanasia

When your gut starts telling you, "It is time," talk to your veterinarian about the appropriate next step. Many times, euthanasia is the only humane option. In this procedure, your veterinarian will give your dog an overdose of anesthesia or barbiturate that will relax him and bring about a quick and painless death.

Ask your veterinarian about the best time of day to do this. Often when veterinary clinics are the least busy—usually during the first appointment in the morning or the last one at night—they can provide the most privacy. Or you might be able to arrange for the veterinarian to come to your house to do the procedure.

You will also have to choose whether or not you want to be present. Keep in mind that it might upset your dog to see you extremely distraught.

You also will have to decide what to do with your dog's remains. Your dog can be cremated with other animals or cremated individually, in which case her ashes can be returned to you. Or you may choose to bury your dog in a pet cemetery or—if permitted by local zoning laws—in your backyard.

Bereavement Support and Counseling

Losing your dog is similar to losing any other family member, so give yourself permission to grieve and seek support if you're not feeling better in a few weeks. There are many pet bereavement and support groups, so don't hesitate to ask your veterinarian for suggestions.

Here are some resources you may find helpful:

- The American Society for the Prevention of Cruelty to Animals' (ASPCA) Pet Loss Hotline: 800-946-4646; enter the PIN number 140-7211 and then add your own phone number. You will be contacted by an ASPCA counselor.
- The Association of Pet Loss and Bereavement: *www.aplb.org*
- Your state's veterinary school for information on local support groups.

Prevent Injuries, Avoid Illnesses and Keep Your Family Safe...You Can Do It!

With the American Red Cross Safety Series, Everything You Need is at Your Fingertips.

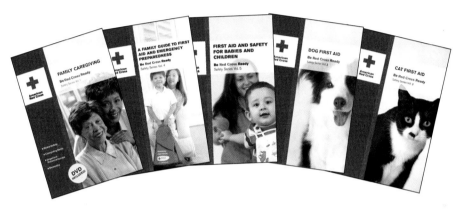

Helping Your Family and Your Community Stay Safe Just Got Easier.

The American Red Cross Safety Series makes it easy to help your family, friends and neighbors stay safe. These easy-to-read guides are designed to help you find information quickly in the event of an emergency. Each one features full color photos and a DVD that helps you and your family build skills even faster. Plus, the guides were developed by the Red Cross, in consultation with leading experts, so you know this is information you can trust.

The Red Cross Safety Series includes these important topics:
• Family Caregiving
• A Family Guide to First Aid and Emergency Preparedness
• First Aid and Safety for Babies and Children
• Dog First Aid
• Cat First Aid

Complete Your Safety Series Today– Visit www.redcross.org/store.

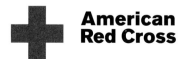

American Red Cross

you can't stop a hurricane.

you can't predict an earthquake.

you can't control a thunderstorm.

but you can be ready.

Visit www.redcross.org

Check out our interactive **Be Red Cross Ready** presentation, then visit *www.redcross.org/store* to find a variety of products and resources to help you be more prepared.

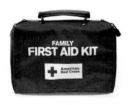

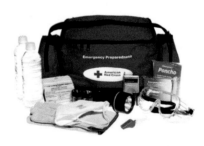

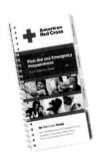

Be Red Cross Ready

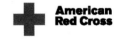